ALLE ZEIT WACH
1842

Claus Claussen Bernd Lochner

Dynamic Computed Tomography

Basic Principles and Clinical Applications

Translated by Frank C. Dougherty

With a Foreword by Roland Felix

With 72 Figures

Springer-Verlag
Berlin Heidelberg New York Tokyo 1985

Priv.-Doz. Dr. med. CLAUS CLAUSSEN
Radiologische Klinik und Poliklinik
Universitätsklinikum Charlottenburg
der Freien Universität
Spandauer Damm 130
D-1000 Berlin 19

Dr. med. BERND LOCHNER
Arzt für Radiologie
Mainzer Landstraße 191
D-6000 Frankfurt 1

Translator
FRANK C. DOUGHERTY
Cite Joffre 13a
D-1000 Berlin 51

ISBN-13:978-3-642-69735-7 e-ISBN-13978-3-642-69733-3
DOI:10.1007/978-3-642-69733-3

Softcover reprint of the hardcover 1st edition 1985

Typesetting and printing: Beltz Offsetdruck, Hemsbach/Bergstr.
Bookbinding: J. Schäffer OHG, 6718 Grünstadt
2121/3130-543210

Foreword

The authors present their experience in more than seven years of dynamic computed tomography in clinical practice. Time density curves and characteristic examples in specific regions of interest enrich the presentation.

Dynamic computed tomography makes an important contribution to the diagnosis and evaluation of a pathologic process: the demonstration of the dynamics of blood flow within the lesion and surrounding normal tissue. Since both the lesion itself and adjacent normal tissue demonstrate characteristic findings in each circulatory phase, the study provides a large amount of data on the flow of blood and contrast material which facilitate both recognition and differentation of a lesion.

Late studies following administration of a contrast agent allow an estimate of the passage of the contrast medium to the interstitium, which is of diagnostic importance.

Chapters dealing with specific clinical entities also contain useful information on the most appropriate means of contrast agent administration (bolus injection or infusion) as well as a discussion of indications for the procedure. Dynamic computed tomography represents a significant advance over conventional computed tomography in some situations, and this signifies a major contribution to the diagnostic capabilities of the clinical radiologist.

The authors are to be commended for the fact that they have clearly defined the limits of dynamic computed tomography. I hope that the first English language edition, following the appearance of the German version in 1983, will be well received.

May 1984 Roland Felix

Preface

Clinical application of computed tomography has reached a developmental plateau since its introduction in 1975. For precisely this reason a large number of textbooks dealing with the clinical use of computed tomography have appeared in the last few years.
Application of contrast material provides greater diagnostic accuracy in many situations. This was immediately apparent after the introduction of tomography, especially in the diagnosis of intracranial lesions.
An impressive scientific symposium dealing with the use of contrast material in computed tomography took place under the chairmanship of R. Felix, E. Kazner and O. H. Wegener in Berlin in 1981. A large number of participants from the United States and Europe emphasized the significance of contrast media in demonstration of individual organs and anatomic regions. Continued developments in CT systems, especially reduced scanning time and increased scan frequency, have been reported in a number of publications dealing with dynamic computed tomography in recent years. We have attempted to develop a survey of the diagnostic possibilities inherent in dynamic computed tomography of the major organs and anatomic regions. Dynamic computed tomography with a third generation CT system has been used in studies of more than 1,500 patients in the Radiology Department of Klinikum Charlottenburg, Free University of Berlin, since Januar 1980. The authors' experience with whole body computed tomography is grounded in 8 years of clinical practice, which began in Heidelberg in 1976 with a 2.5-min device.

Claus Claussen,
Bernd Lochner

Contents

1 Introduction

The high density resolution of computed tomography (CT) allows demonstration of structures within parenchymal organs and determinations of differences in density in these structures. However, circumscribed lesions may go undetected if they are small or if there is only a slight difference in density as compared with surrounding tissues. The size of a demonstrable lesion is a function of its density. For example, it is possible to demonstrate a small calcified lesion 1 mm in diameter within the liver, while tumors measuring several centimeters are not visible if their density is only slightly different from that of surrounding tissue and if the lesions have caused no visible alterations in normal structures.

Intravenous application of contrast media is standard practice in CT studies for clarification of intracranial lesions, especially brain tumors, since disruption of the blood-brain barrier results in pathologic contrast enhancement in many tumors. This may provide the first indication of the presence of a lesion. In addition, the degree of contrast enhancement provides useful information in differentiation among a number of diagnostic possibilities.

The role of contrast media in CT studies of the abdominal organs was not well defined in the early phases of whole body scanning, since the indications for administration of contrast material were not as clearly defined as those in cranial CT. For example, some authors maintained that contrast administration was unnecessary in the diagnosis of space-occupying hepatic lesions.

The development of CT systems with scan times of several seconds resulted in considerable improvement in picture quality as well as reduction in artifacts due to patient motion. As a result, a number of investigators began to probe the viability of contrast enhancement in CT in order to test the applicability of contrast studies in various clinical situations.

An increase in the density gradient between a circumscribed lesion and surrounding normal tissue results in improved demonstration of details, a major factor in the use of contrast media.

Dynamic CT meets the requirement of recording a large number of images within the shortest possible time and attempts to define both morphological and functional characteristics of an organ. To this purpose, contrast material is administered and images are recorded in rapid succession within a single slice. The dynamics of contrast enhancement are then evaluated. This requires a large number of images in a short period, quantitative evaluation, and simple, variable, and reproducible operating conditions. Short scan times and high scan frequency allow documentation and evaluation of the dynamics of contrast enhancement, especially in the initial phase of contrast uptake after bolus administration. Time-density measurements allow quantitative evaluation.

Time-dependent changes in density following contrast administration permit evaluation of organ function and provide information on the nature of pathologic processes. Dynamic CT requires rapid bolus injection, and this limits the choice of contrast material to water-soluble substances with renal elimination. Contrast agents cleared by the liver and biliary tract generally demonstrate high toxicity as a result of significant plasma protein binding, and rapid application of these substances results in higher toxicity.

Continuous intravenous administration of a contrast agent results in better contrast in many CT applications. However, dynamic CT studies are not possible with this mode of contrast administration except in cardiac studies, and these applications will therefore be dealt with only in passing in this book.

Both noninvasive dynamic CT and digital substraction angiography analyze the distribution of contrast media in the vascular bed after bolus administration. It is of particular interest to define the time and duration of maximum contrast enhancement in order to achieve the greatest possible increase in density gradient between the vascular system and the initial low contrast values in the extravascular space. Demonstration of contrast material in the vascular bed is the primary consideration in dynamic CT within the first minute after contrast administration. As in conventional angiography, CT studies demonstrate vascular relations and the passage of contrast media to the capillary bed, which is defined as the "parenchymal phase" in conventional angiography. Demonstration of contrast enhancement in the extravascular space is important in later phases, as a number of authors noted in earlier studies with slower CT systems. Reports in the literature are not as yet conclusive on the means for obtaining optimal contrast enhancement. Controversy continues on the types of contrast material, dosages, and mode of injection.

The theoretical portion of this book (Chaps. 1–5) deals with the factors influencing the degree and duration of contrast enhancement in the vascular bed and major organs. In addition, time-density measurements will be presented to describe the initial vascular phase and subsequent diffusion and distribution of contrast material in the extravascular space.

In Chap. 6, which deals with clinical applications, density measurements in disease processes of various organs will be demonstrated, and characteristic contrast enhancement in dynamic CT studies of specific organ lesions discussed.

2 Basic Physical Principles and Technical Considerations

2.1 Attenuation Coefficients

Attenuation of X-rays as they pass through material is determined by a number of interrelationships, such as photoelectric absorption and the Compton effect. Attenuation within biological tissue is a function of chemical composition, density, X-ray filtration, and voltage in the X-ray system. The following equation describes the attenuation of X-rays in a given medium, with I_0 the initial intensity of the X-ray beam, d the thickness of the medium and I the resulting intensity:

$$I = I_0 e^{-(\mu E d)}$$

This holds true for radiation of the energy E in a homogeneous medium. μE is the linear attenuation coefficient of radiation with energy E. An increase in thickness or an increase in the linear attenuation coefficient entails a corresponding reduction in the resulting radiation intensity I. There is an inverse relationship between the linear attenuation coefficient and radiation energy such that higher energy results in a lower linear attenuation coefficient. The latter is determined from a number of measured values at defined angles for each element of the picture. As a result, μ is an empirical value which depends on the size, shape, and composition of an object and which may be considered as an attenuation value associated with a given energy level.

Attenuation coefficients for soft tissues in the human body approximate those of water. Bone tissue has an attenuation coefficient nearly double that of water, while air has such a low density that its attenuation coefficient is negligible. In 1972 Hounsfield established a scale for density determinations in human tissue based on linear attenuation coefficients. The scale gives relative attenuation coefficients which are termed density values. These CT units were named Hounsfield units (HU) after the innovator of CT and defined as follows:

$$\text{CT values (HU)} = 1000 \frac{\mu_x - \mu_{H_2O}}{\mu_{H_2O}}$$

The density (μ) of water is zero, that of air −1000, and that of solid bone +1000 HU. Fat tissue is approximately −100 HU, while most organs with soft tissue density have values between 30 and 80 HU.

2.2 Mathematical Picture Reconstruction

A major advantage of CT over conventional radiological techniques is the fact that overlying and neighboring structures are eliminated, which allows accurate representation of the organ structures within the plane in question. Tomographic studies without superposition of adjacent structures is possible primarily as a result of the reconstruction process used in CT. The X-ray detectors register values which represent attenuation values in the plane, and these values are processed in order to provide a visual display. Mathematical processing permits calculation of a two-dimensional distribution of CT values on the basis of attenuation profiles.

2.3 Attenuation Values and Visual Displays

The X-ray beam is attenuated according to known physical laws by interaction with electrons at every point along its path within a tissue. Attenuation is a function of energy of the X-ray beam, the physical density ϱ, and the effective atomic number of the tissue. Hübener (1978) demonstrated "an approximately linear relationship between the absorption value μ and the physical density ϱ of a given point" within soft tissues at constant voltages.

Values obtained at given points are processed in the computer, stored in the quadratic matrix according to their attenuation values, transferred to a visual matrix with identical capacity, and displayed on a television monitor with the help of an analog gray scale. Earlier systems used a matrix with 160×160 points while most modern systems use a matrix of 256×256 picture elements ("pixels"). Processing takes place in a high-speed calculator which analyzes incoming data in three separate consecutive steps during the scanning procedure, and the visual display appears on the monitor as soon as the scan is terminated.

Absorption values are expressed in terms of density on the Hounsfield scale and demonstrated visually as gradations on a gray scale comprising 16 steps, each representing 16 density values. Measured density is displayed in Hounsfield units. Visual demonstration of the density values on a gray scale is limited by the capacity of the human eye to discriminate among a maximum of 20 gradations of gray. However, shifting or widening the spectrum of attenuation values at a given point on the density scale allows optimal demonstration of all attenuation values of diagnostic interest with the gray scale.

2.4 Criteria of Picture Quality

As a result of limited scatter radiation and elimination of superimposed structures, CT studies permit high resolution of objects with low radiologic contrast. This is decisive in the diagnosis of soft tissue lesions. Spatial resolution is an additional important criterion of picture quality.

Spatial resolving power is defined by the size of structures which can be differentiated with high contrast. This, in turn, is dependent on the resolving power of the system and the thickness of the tomographic slice in question. Thickness of the slice is defined as half the width of the sensitivity profile perpendicular to the plane in the middle of the field. In a relatively thick slice, such as 8 mm, all X-rays passing through the object are registered by the detector and utilized for construction of the visual image. The dose profile corresponds to the sensitivity profile. In very thin slices – e. g. 2 mm – the X-rays must be carefully focused by means of aperture controls on the X-ray tube and the detector in order to limit scatter radiation. The advantage of thin slices lies in the high specificity of demonstration within the slice, since thicker slices necessarily include a number of structures and interference may result.

There is an evident interrelationship between spatial and density resolution, both of which determine the picture quality of CT studies. Spatial resolution depends primarily on the distribution of the detectors, while density resolution depends on the spatial distribution of density values, the radiation dose, and the procedure used for reconstruction of the image. In addition, Schultz and Felix (1978) demonstrated that other factors, such as the shape and distribution of objects in the slice, may influence picture quality.

Contrast or density resolution defines the diameter of an object which can be differentiated from surrounding structures at low contrast levels. In practice, this defines the size and density of a lesion which can be recognized and differentiated from adjacent tissue. The contrast between two different tissues is defined as the difference in CT values:

$$\Delta CT\ 1,2 = CT_2 - CT_1$$

The contrast between the highest and lowest values in a slice is defined by two terms, modulation depth and relative contrast, which is approximately double the modulation depth. Picture quality in reconstructed CT studies is determined by contrast within an object and depends on radiation dose, distribution of energy at the detector, and sensitivity of the detector system.

Image noise and the size of the object under study are limiting factors. Measurement of density values requires registration of an adequate minimum number of X-ray quantums, which is achieved by repeated measurements. The signals received by all detectors represent a given signal amplitude, which varies about a mean value. This area of variability about a single measurement is termed signal noise. Signal strength and noise must remain within limits if adequate resolution is to be achieved. As a result, the contrast sensitivity of CT depends primarily on quantum noise. At given volumes and known quantum values it is possible to establish limits for quantum noise which are a function of slice thickness, pixel size, and radiation dose.

A large radiation dose or an object with limited attenuation decreases noise. For example, it is possible to reduce pixel noise by a factor of 2 when dosage is increased 4 times. On the other hand, reduction of pixel size by half requires a corresponding eightfold increase in radiation dose in order to maintain the same relationship between signal strength and noise. In addition, the digital nature of the visual display limits spatial resolution.

2.5 Spatial Resolution and Discrimination at High Contrast Levels

Determinations of high contrast resolution are made with a high contrast Plexiglas phantom. A round Plexiglas plate 20 cm in diameter contains a row of holes of different diameters arranged in such a way that the midpoints of adjacent holes are equal to twice the diameter of the holes themselves. The largest hole measures 4 mm in diameter, the smallest 0.5 mm. The studies are made with slices of various thicknesses, with different radiation doses at a constant voltage of 125 kV and varying mAs, and with different zoom factors. Resolution is defined as the row in which adjacent holes are demonstrated as clearly separate from one another.

The best resolution in our series was achieved with a slice thickness of 2 mm, a zoom factor of 4, voltage at 125 kV, 460 mAs, and an exposure time of 10 s with the convolution kernel 1 "Body" and 720 projections. With the Siemens Somatom 2 system it is possible to demonstrate objects as small as 0.9 mm as separate objects. Reducing the distance between the objects results in overlapping of their absorption profiles, and the naked eye is not able to discriminate between the adjacent objects. When the parameters defined above are used with a slice thickness of 8 mm, adjacent objects measuring 0.9 mm are still demonstrated as separate entities. However, resolving power is significantly reduced when a zoom factor of 2 is used, and a diameter of 1.25 mm is the limit of resolution. Newer CT systems with high resolution programs are capable of demonstrating objects as small as 0.6 mm. This is useful for examining small structures in the middle and internal ear, such as the ossicles.

Resolution is considerably reduced at 360 projections and 230 mAs. A zoom factor of 1.7 is usually used in dynamic CT studies, which allows resolution of objects 1.5 mm in diameter. Our studies have shown that spatial resolution is independent of dosage at higher contrast levels: spatial resolution is identical at 230 mAs and 460 mAs when slice thickness, convolution kernel and number of projections are identical.

2.6 Spatial Resolution at Low Contrast Levels

Determinations of spatial resolution at low contrast levels are made using a polyethylene phantom with rows of holes of different diameters. The distance between midpoints of two adjacent holes in a row is equal to twice the diameter of the holes, which range from 1 to 40 mm in diameter in the most commonly used phantoms. The holes are filled with an alcohol solution, which results in a defined contrast to the polyethylene phantom.

Even when differences in density are as low as 4 HU, it is possible to discriminate between holes 6 mm in diameter with slice thicknesses of 8 mm and 460 mAs (Fig. 1b). With 720 projections, 460 mAs, 8-mm slices, and contrast of 40 HU it is possible to discriminate between holes measuring 1.25 mm in diameter (Fig. 1a). Contrast resolution is significantly lower with slice thicknesses of 2 mm:

Fig. 1a–c. Spatial resolution at different contrast levels. **a** Resolution with contrast ΔHU 40, 8-mm slice, 720 projections, 460 mAs, 125 kV, zoom factor 2. **b** Resolution at low contrast levels (ΔHU 4), 8-mm slice, 720 projections, 460 mAs, 125 kV, zoom factor 2. **c** 2-mm slice with poorer resolution and increased noise

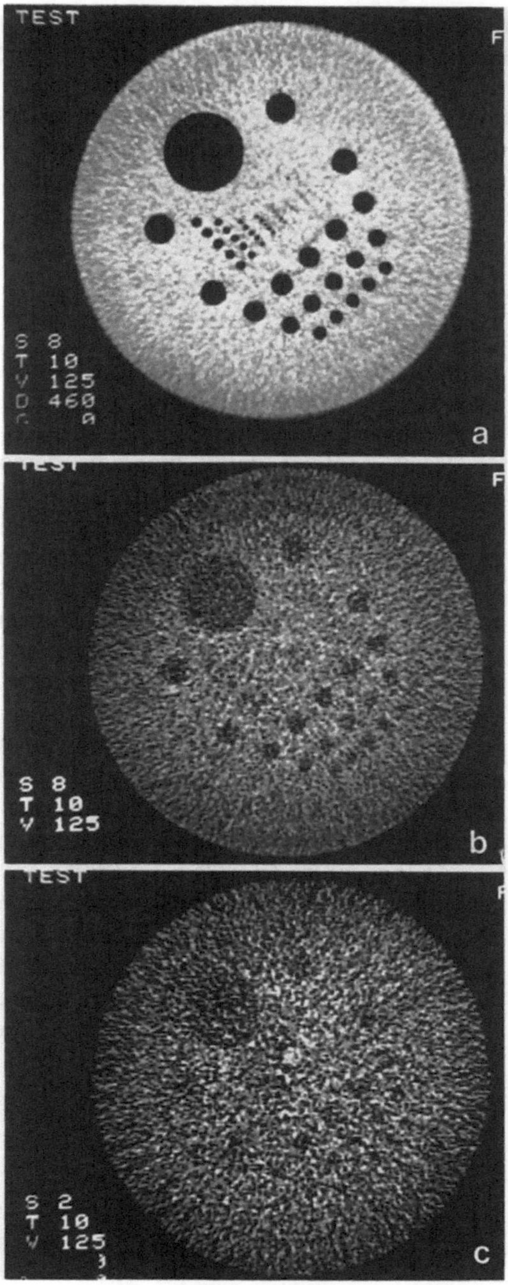

maximum resolution is 10 mm with 720 projections and 460 mAs (Fig. 1c). The limit of contrast resolution with density differences of 40 HU is 2 mm in diameter.

The reason for poor contrast resolution with 2-mm slices as compared with 8-mm slices is stronger noise, which results in poorer contrast resolution with thinner slices at a given dosage level in the low contrast region. Higher contrast resolution can only be achieved with higher radiation doses.

2.7 Contrast Detail Diagrams

Determinations of spatial resolution with high contrast and low contrast phantoms at various slice thicknesses, projections, and zoom factors are recorded on double logarithmic scales.

These contrast detail diagrams demonstrate the limits of both spatial resolution and contrast resolution for objects of a given size. The limit of resolution at high contrast levels is parallel to the y-axis. This shows that high contrast resolution, necessary for demonstration of bone structures, is greatest in thin slices (2 mm), at 460 mAs, 720 projections, and exposure of 10 s. Spatial resolution is not increased at zoom factors greater than 4. Contrast resolution for soft tissue structures is found in the lower portion of the curve and approaches the x-axis asymptotically. Small structures require high contrast to their surroundings (Fig. 2a, b).

The diameters of objects demonstrated with a CT system are found to the right and above the curve; the contrast detail relationships to the left and below the curve escape demonstration. Contrast detail diagrams consequently define the limits for demonstration of objects at different contrast levels.

At low contrast levels CT systems are superior to conventional radiologic techniques in demonstration of objects larger than 1 mm in diameter. However, resolution of small details well below 1 mm in diameter with high contrast is possible with conventional radiologic techniques but not with CT.

Dynamic CT studies made with a slice thickness of 8 mm, 230 mAs, and 125 kV provide adequate contrast resolution and are superior to studies made with 2 mm slices, since contrast resolution is decisive in this technique.

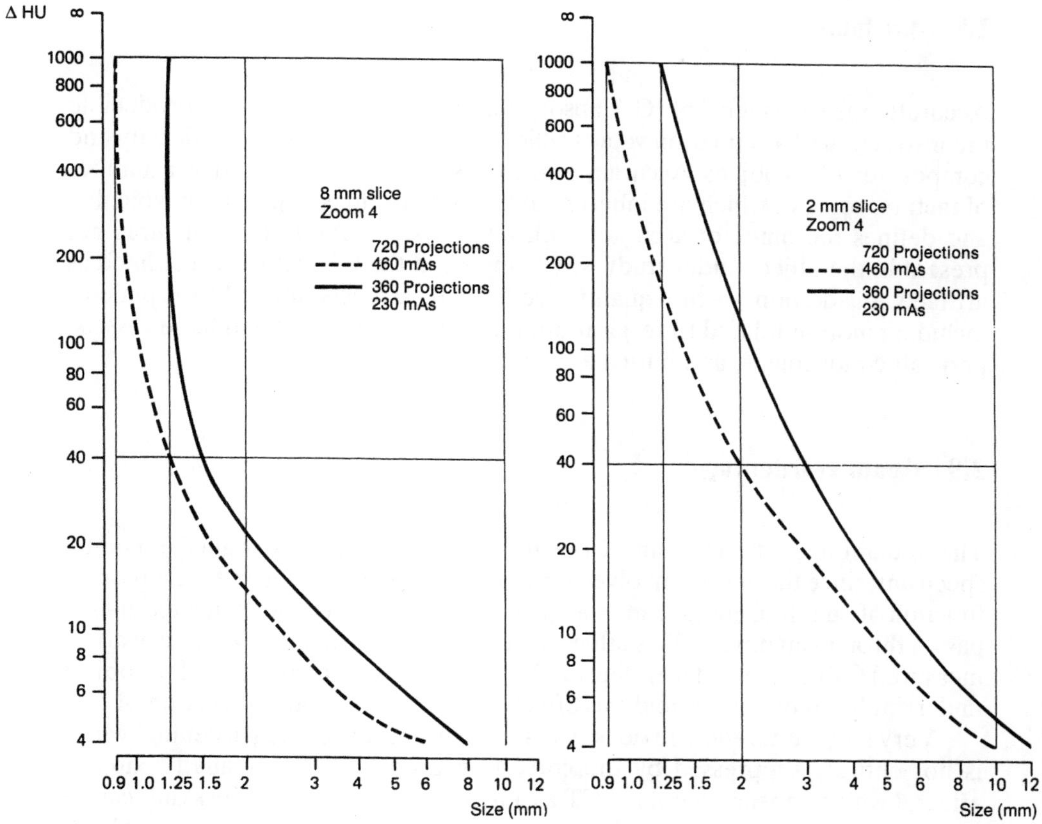

Fig. 2a, b. Contrast detail diagrams

2.8 Artifacts

Accurate measurement of CT absorption values depends on reproducible reconstruction of attenuation values which, in turn, are a function of density and composition of an object. Accuracy of the CT study may be reduced by a number of factors, some of which are inherent in the system. Image noise is unavoidable and defines the limits of accuracy with a CT system. All other structures not present in the object under study which appear in the CT picture are defined as artifacts. In addition, picture quality is reduced by artifacts caused by the patient, including motion related to respiration, pulsation of the heart and large vessels, peristaltic movement, and muscular contraction.

2.9 Beam Hardening

The radiation emitted by an X-ray tube is defined as a so-called quantum spectrum, since the energy involved is not uniform. Attenuation coefficients are a function of quantum energy, and the quantum spectrum changes when the energy passes through an object. This effect is termed beam hardening, which can affect measured CT numbers, depending on the attenuation characteristics of the object under study. In order to avoid this effect, CT systems contain correction filters.

Very large differences in density result in disproportionate hardening, which is not entirely suppressed by the correction process. The so-called "cupping effect," which appears in cranial CT as a hyperdense zone near the skull, can be avoided by use of special convolution kernels. Hardening may appear near bone structures as well as around blood vessels containing contrast media. The effect is especially common in dynamic CT studies, since the latter often demonstrate wide ranges of density values after contrast enhancement. False density values up to ± 10 HU secondary to beam hardening may also be found in large abdominal organs such as the liver and spleen near the ribs, as Schultz and Lackner demonstrated in measurements on phantoms (1981).

2.10 Partial Volume Effect

When a given slice contains structures with extreme density values such as bone or air, inhomogeneity may cause effects such as lines, stripes, or rings similar to beam hardening, which may result in inaccurate measurements. So-called partial volume effects occur when a structure surpasses a given slice, with the result that false density values are measured. The source of this error lies in the fact that each element within the slice is treated as a homogeneous structure, and objects with various density values within a given volume are represented by mean density values in the reconstructed image. Structures with a wide range of density values, such as the base of the skull, are examined with thin slices of 2 or 4 mm in order to eliminate this effect.

Errors may also result from an inadequate number of measurements within a single projection or from an inadequate number of projections. These result in so-called aliasing errors in objects with sharp borders and high contrast, such as the base of the skull. Doubling the number of projections to 720 may compensate for these errors. The latter are not found in the upper abdomen, where transitions in density values are more gradual. The number of necessary projections is also a function of the size of the field and frequency of the modulation transfer function. More projections are necessary in a larger field and at higher frequencies. At 360 projections, filters are necessary at the limits of the field in order to provide adequate measurements in soft tissue studies, and it is essential that the entire patient be within the field.

2.11 Radiation Dose

In modern CT systems the X-ray tube revolves around the patient and exposes an extremely narrow field. This reduces scatter radiation, with the result that structures adjacent to the slice are exposed to considerably less radiation than with conventional radiologic techniques. Radiation distribution on the body surface is the algebraic sum of incident and transmitted radiation. Movement of the X-ray tube around the body results in a series of impulses from 360 positions, which produces a fairly even dose on the skin surface. At a constant voltage of 125 kV the absorbed dose is a function of mAs product and the number of projections in each scan. Thermoluminescence instruments located within phantoms with absorption characteristics similar to the human body, such as the Alderson phantom, allow measurements of radiation dose distribution within the body and demonstrate practically symmetrical isodose curves with CT systems using 360° revolution.

At 125 kV and 230 mAs maximum skin dose is 12.5 mGy (1.25 rad) with the Somatom 2, and this value is independent of exposure, number of projections, and thickness of slice. Skin dose is proportional to the mAs product, and the skin dose at 460 mAs is double that at 230 mAs.

The length-dose product – the integral of the dosage profile along a line perpendicular to the slice at various levels within the phantom – is useful for calculating dose in adjacent slices and at various depths. There is a clear relationship to slice thickness. When a large number of adjacent slices are registered, the skin dose is the quotient of the length-dose product at the surface and the thickness of the slice.

CT studies of the body made with an 8-mm slice at 230 mAs and 125 kV result in a surface dose of 20.5 mGy (2.05 rad) at a superficial length-dose product of 16.4 mGy/cm. When 2-mm slices are made with 460 mAs – for demonstration of intervertebral disks, for example – the dose is 50 mGy (5 rad).

Dose distribution within a CT slice with the Somatom 2 was measured with a 20-cm Plexiglas phantom rather than with the Alderson phantom. It is possible to calculate dose distribution in a given slice when the length-dose product is divided by slice thickness (Table 1).

Table 1. Dose at 125 kV, 230 mAs; 8-mm slice

Depth (cm)	Dose (mGy)
0	16.4 : 0.8 = 20.5
1	16.6 : 0.8 = 20.75
3.6	15.3 : 0.8 = 19.13
10.0	13.1 : 0.8 = 16.38

Approximate dose values for a single study can be obtained by multiplying these values by the quotient of the dose within a single slice and the dose from multiple slices at the surface:

$$\frac{12.5\ \text{mGy}}{20.5\ \text{mGy}} = 0.61$$

Mean organ dose is calculated on the assumption of linear relationships between dose and radiation effects in the organ exposed to radiation. Total dose is the sum of direct radiation exposure within each slice and scatter radiation. Dose to the gonads depends on the distance between the body region under study and the gonads themselves; the values cited above apply in cases of direct exposure.

3 Dynamic Computed Tomography

3.1 Technical Considerations

Dynamic CT allows measurements of temporal changes in contrast density after bolus administration of contrast material. Changes in density are registered in the blood vessels and in soft tissues.

Prerequisites for dynamic studies are short scan time, short scan intervals, high scan frequency, and a large total number of scans. Dynamic CT has also been termed sequence CT and serial CT since a number of scans are made in series within a single slice.

Considerable flexibility is also required for serial CT studies, since rapid sequences may be followed by scans at longer and variable intervals. In addition, quantitative evaluation and relative simplicity of operation are required. Resolution in dynamic CT studies must be as high as that achieved by conventional CT, since demonstration of slight changes in density within tissues following contrast administration is an absolute prerequisite for dynamic CT. Registration of slight differences in density is possible only at low noise levels, since the limit for demonstration of differences in density is directly proportional to noise.

In addition, mechanical instability may cause errors in dynamic CT studies. The X-ray tube and the detector system are mounted on a metal ring and move around the patient. The technical elements are accelerated, decelerated, and accelerated once again in the opposite direction during the procedure (Figs. 3, 4). The centrifugal forces which develop may contribute to mechanical instability of the CT apparaturs.

The X-ray tube itself is the major limiting factor, since it determines scan time, frequency, and contrast resolution. High resolution is currently attainable only with large mAs products, i.e. at high radiation doses. A large number of scans in rapid succession places considerable strain on the X-ray tube as a result of the limited capacity of the anode for storing heat energy. This limits the number of scans that can be recorded in rapid succession. Reduction of the mAs product requires prolonged scan times. In summary, the X-ray tube is the limiting factor in determining scan frequency and contrast resolution.

Modern CT systems allow automation of the scanning process with preselection of the number and frequency of scans.

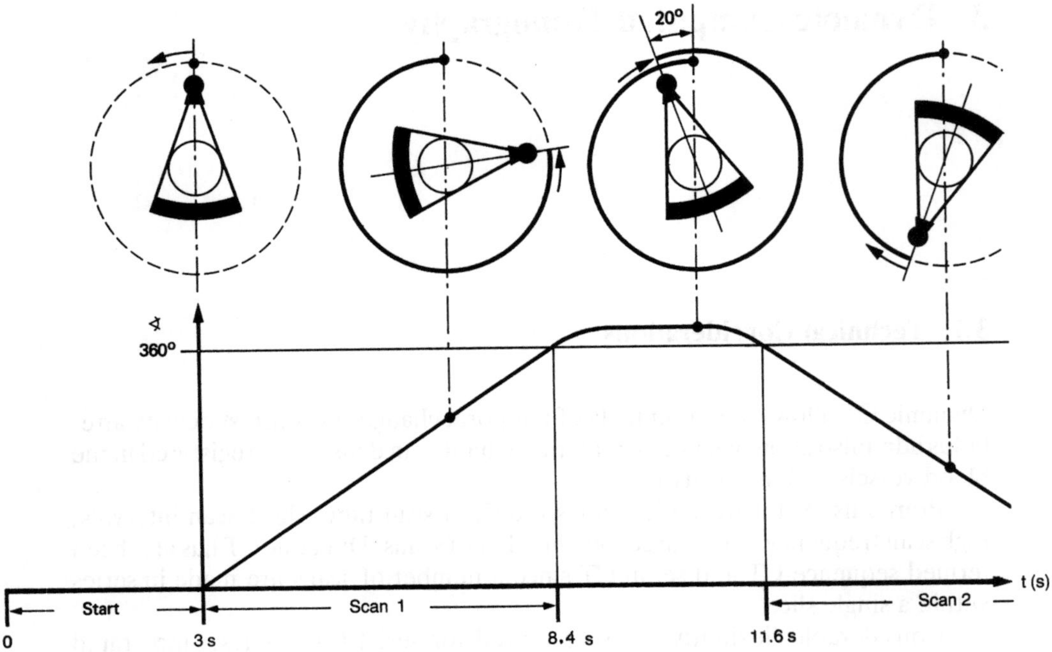

Fig. 3. Movement of the X-ray tube and the detector system at maximum scan frequency (7/min)

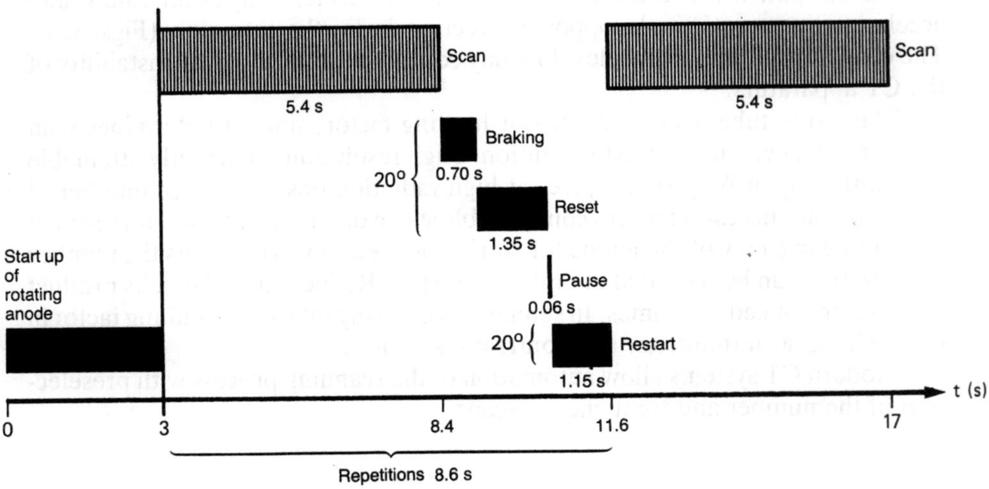

Fig. 4. Temporal relations in a scan with a third generation system (7 scans/min)

3.2 Scan Splitting

The limitations on scan time and frequency described above led to the development of segmental picture reconstruction. With the Somatom 2 three 240° pictures can be reconstructed from a normal 360° scan, which provides information on changes in density during the 360° scan procedure. Weighting factors ranging from 0 to 1 are necessary to eliminate artifacts which develop when the data obtained at the limit of the scan sector are used for split reconstructions. The split images are based on data obtained in a sector measuring 240° with corrections made at the limits of the 240° sector (Fig. 5). Since the original data are obtained over 360°, and there is no overlapping between 0 and 360°, the data recorded at 0° are artificially underrepresented in split reconstructions. The results of split reconstruction and 360° reconstruction are never identical in studies of objects which change over time, as is the case in density changes following administration of contrast material.

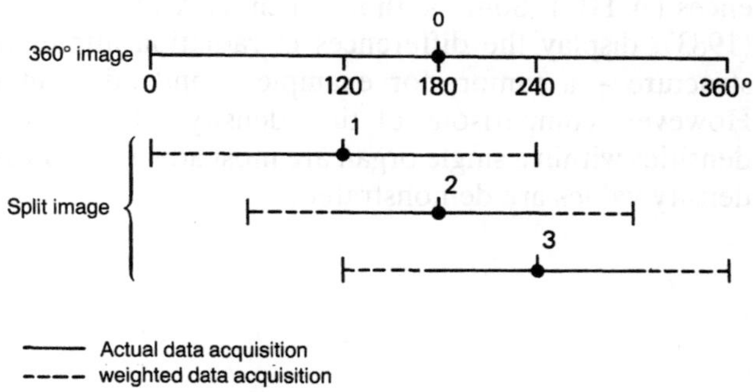

Fig. 5. Data acquisition in multiphase reconstruction

3.3 Time-Density Measurements

Quantitative evaluation of density within a tissue is possible at any given point or area in a CT picture. A number of programs allow density measurements at given points, circular areas, or defined regions – so-called "regions of interest" (ROI) – of any desired size. Mean attenuation values and standard deviation are determined within these areas and demonstrated in the CT picture. It is possible to measure density at any given point within the picture.

Changes in density over time after intravenous application of contrast material can be demonstrated in a series of CT pictures made at short intervals.

A separate program analyzes time-density relations in freely selected ROIs and demonstrates the results in time-density diagrams (Fig. 6). In addition, it is possible to determine mean density values and standard deviations for each CT picture within a scan series. The increase in density after contrast enhancement is more evident when the values registered in the plain scan are subtracted from density values measured after contrast application, resulting in density differences (Δ HU). Some authors, such as Araki et al. (1980) and Majewski et al. (1983), display the differences in radiation attenuation between a pathologic structure – a tumor, for example – and adjacent normal tissue over time. However, comparisons of time-density relations in structures with different densities within a single organ are most advantageously presented when absolute density values are demonstrated.

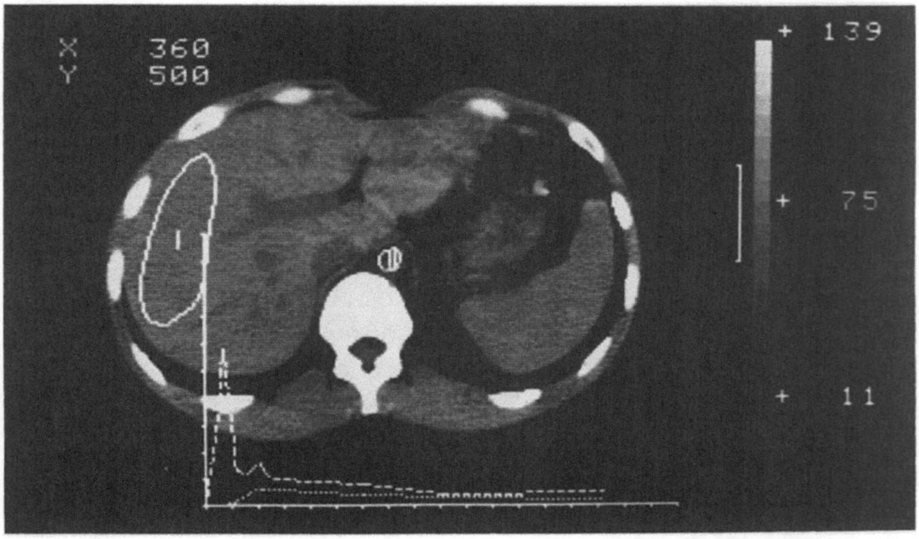

Fig. 6. Regions of interest in the aorta and liver with time-density diagrams following intravenous injection of a contrast agent (60 ml, flow rate 8 ml/s). x-axis = 360 s; y-axis = 500 HU

3.4 ECG-Triggered Cardiac CT Studies

Serial CT studies are also used to demonstrate changes in distribution of contrast material over time in the heart, e. g. for demonstration of aortocoronary bypass graft patency or myocardial perfusion over time.

However, it is practically impossible to make density measurements in a moving object such as the heart with scan times from 1 to 5 s, as is the case with modern CT systems. The latter use ECG-triggered techniques to demonstrate the heart in various phases of the cardiac cycle.

A single scan period of 1–5 s necessarily includes several cardiac cycles, with the result that the contours developed in the computer of the CT system are blurred due to motion artifacts. Delineation of individual segments of the heart in different portions of the cardiac cycle is often impossible. CT is incapable of registering disorders of regional wall motion in a given phase of the heart cycle unless ECG-triggered cardio-CT systems are used. ECG triggering results in significant improvement in picture quality in heart studies. Identical phases of the cardiac cycle are used for picture reconstruction. However, this implies that not all 360 projections of a single scan are available for picture reconstruction. In order to take advantage of all 360 projections, multiple scans – usually eight in all – are necessary within a single slice. The number of scans necessary is a function of the R–R interval. For example, within R–R intervals of 0.7 s, one picture made in four scans includes a time interval of 0.17 s, as compared with 0.08 s with eight scans.

Each exposure in a series is made by the operator. The computer uses the ECG tracing and identifies projections which have already been recorded and those necessary for a given R–R interval; the data recorded at individual exposures are then collected for picture reconstruction in given phases of the cardiac cycle. After the exposures are made, picture matrices are reconstructed mathematically for the desired phases and intervals. The phases of the cardiac cycle are expressed in percentages such that an entire cardiac cycle or R–R

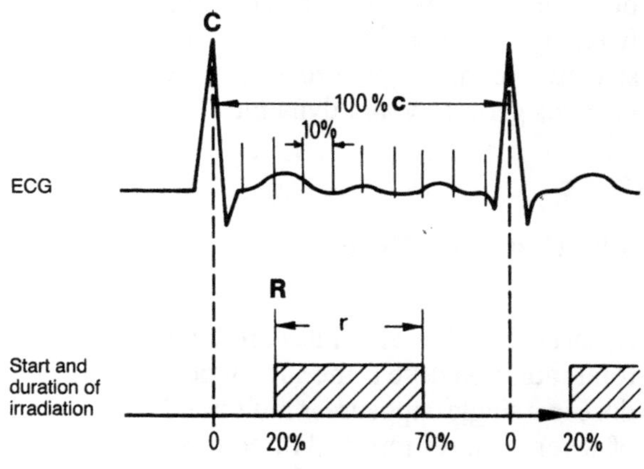

Fig. 7. Example of ECG-triggered cardio-CT study; *C*, start of the cycle; *c*, duration of the cycle; *R*, start of irradiation; *r*, duration of irradiation. The cycle begins at the R wave

interval is equal to 100% (Fig. 7), and the different phases within a given cycle are assigned percentage values. For example, systole lies between 30% and 40% of the R–R interval and diastole between 80% and 90%. These are the moments of relative immobility with the least number of motion artifacts. However, it is not possible to fix the systolic and diastolic endpoints with perfect accuracy, which results in slight imprecision. Individual scans containing motion artifacts contribute nothing to the picture reconstruction and are eliminated.

Cardiac arrhythmias pose a problem for ECG-triggered CT studies since regular sinus rhythm is necessary for control of the CT system. In arrhythmia, the computer receives data from different phases in the cardiac cycle, which renders evaluation and picture reconstruction impossible. ECG-triggered CT studies require a cooperative patient in regular sinus rhythm. In addition, the slices must be made in the same plane, which implies a constant respiratory position.

3.5 Serial Digital Radiography

Kruger et al. (1981) and Hübener et al. (1982) introduced chronography as a procedure for serial digital radiographic studies within a given slice. The method is still experimental. Whereas in digital radiographs the patient is moved on a belt below a fixed X-ray tube, in the chronographic procedure the patient is immobile. A burst of X-ray impulses (40 s) passes through the body in a single plane. After administration of a contrast agent, radiation attenuation is measured within the slice at five selected time intervals up to 1 min. Heart rate, respiration, and voluntary motion change the transmission profile.

Subtraction of the values obtained before contrast administration from those registered in the contrast study permits detection of slight changes in attenuation, since the system has high density resolution.

This technique facilitates determination of the point in time at which a bolus of contrast medium reaches any body region with a given injection technique. In practice, the region is selected and X-ray pulses are delivered at short intervals from a fixed position. The attenuation profiles are displayed so that each structure in the CT picture is assigned a column. The method allows exact studies of bolus geometry and dynamics.

3.6 Radiation Dose

In serial CT several studies are made in the same plane, which implies that the total radiation dose is the sum of doses in the individual exposures. The radiation dose in a single exposure is multiplied by the number of slices. At a scan frequency of seven pictures/min and three slices at different points in time – as is the case in dynamic CT studies –, with a slice thickness of 8 mm at 230 mAs and 125 kV the surface dose is 125 mGy (12.5 rad).

3.7 Future Developments

Kalender (1981) defined the goals of future developments in dynamic CT studies as being:
1. Increased scan rates
2. X-ray tubes with higher performance
3. Simultaneous studies of more than one slice at a time

The following new concepts are theoretically attractive:
1. Multiple X-ray tubes
2. Continuous revolution of the system in one direction

The second idea would eliminate the interval between subsequent scans. These two concepts are currently under study in experimental scanners in the United States.

The systems under study at the Mayo Clinic use the components of current CT systems. Twenty-eight X-ray tubes are mounted in a semicircle across from a semicircular screen backed up by 28 television cameras. The gantry is approximately 4 m in diameter, weighs 15 tons, and reaches a speed of 15 revolutions per second. Sixty pictures per second are possible when the gantry is stationary. The television screen allows demonstration of entire organs rather than single slices. However, major problems have been encountered. The dynamics of the screen are relatively limited, scatter radiation is considerable, and problems have developed with the reconstruction algorithm. The gantry is stationary, with the result that less than 180° are registered, and the problem of reconstruction of multiple slices from exposures using divergent beams has still to be solved.

The second concept has been realized in an experimental scanner for cardiac studies in use at the University of California at San Francisco. In place of conventional X-ray tubes revolving around the patient, this system employs a 220° anode ring across from a stationary 220° detector ring. An electron beam emanating from the cathode is eletromagnetically focused on the entire anode after passage through a vacuum. This system contains no moving parts, and scan times as short as 25 ms without dead intervals between the scans have been achieved. However, the anode and detector rings overlap to a certain extent, and the slices are not uniformly exposed. Artifacts have imposed serious limitations on quantitative evaluation.

3.8 Examination Techniques and Evaluation

The CT studies are made with the patient in the supine position. Dynamic CT studies are made with a scan frequency of six scans/min with a total of nine scans. Six scans are made in the first minute, with individual scans at 120, 180, and 300 s after bolus injection of contrast material. The physician remains with the patient during the scanning procedure in order to perform the injection, to start the CT series, and to instruct the patient to hold his breath. The scan is made in expiratory apnea. The patient takes one deep breath in each interval between scans during the first minute. Most patients are able to tolerate rapid contrast administration and repeated apnea with this technique.

Initial plain scans of the abdomen are made and the slice for the serial CT studies selected. Slice thickness is 8 mm and voltage 125 kV at 230 mAs.

The contrast medium is injected at the cubital vein using a 16 G or 14 G Abocath which allows contrast administration at rates up to 12 ml/s.

A flow-directed injector is used for dynamic CT studies. This results in standardized and reproducible conditions for administration of contrast agents. The latter are warmed to 37°C before administration. We use an injection rate of 8 ml/s for standard dynamic CT studies.

Meglumine diatrizoate (Angiografin, Schering) containing 30 mg iodine per milliliter – or, in more recent studies, iohexal (Omnipaque) – is used for serial CT studies. Total volume of contrast material administered is a function of body weight, with 1 ml/kg body weight as the usual dose.

Time-density measurements are made in regions of interest such as the liver, the spleen, the kidneys, the abdominal aorta, the vena cava, and suspected pathologic structures. The regions of interest are defined as large as possible in order to avoid errors resulting from small volumes. Measurements in the liver are made in areas without large blood vessels. Mean density values are determined at defined points in time within each region of interest. Standard deviation of ± 5% is acceptable in regions of interest in the liver and spleen. Standard deviation in the density measurements following contrast administration is only slightly higher than the values obtained in plain scans of the liver and spleen. This compares with significantly higher standard deviations of up to 10% in the aorta following administration of contrast agents.

Changes in density are evaluated with a computer program. In order to assure that each region of interest in the series is identical and not altered by respiratory motion or artifacts in the CT system, each measurement is checked and documented. After calibration, measurements should be made on a water phantom in order to calculate standard deviation at water density (0 HU) before dynamic CT studies are made. Standard deviations $\varrho = 0.5\%$ or ± 5 HU are possible as a result of the statistical variation of the energy in the X-ray tube, and variations in density values of ± 5 HU are tolerated. This variation becomes less significant in large regions of interest, and evaluation of density measurements should include at least four or five points within a single field. Density values derived from a single measurement at a single point should not be used for quantitative evaluation. Interpolation procedures allow enlargements of defined segments of the CT picture. However, this is simply a process of optical enlargement and does not furnish new density measurements.

Evaluation of small structures is facilitated when certain enlargement factors are used in order to attain smaller standard deviations in some density measurements.

In some cases time-density curves are used for demonstration of typical changes in density following contrast administration (Fig. 6). For purposes of comparison, increases in density after contrast enhancement can be readily expressed as time-density curves using the differences between density values in the plain scan and the contrast study (Δ HU).

4 Contrast Media

Use of substances with high radiologic density for the demonstration of blood vessels and organs has been part of clinical routine in conventional radiology for decades. The high atomic numbers of these positive contrast agents such as iodine and barium increase attentuation of X-rays within the human body.

4.1 Types of Contrast Media

Water-soluble contrast media based on triiodobenzene are most often used in dynamic CT studies.

The dimeric contrast media used in studies of the biliary tract have strong protein binding and cannot be administered rapidly by the i. v. route for dynamic CT studies, because rapid application would increase the incidence of side-effects. The maximum increase in density within the liver is only 10–15 HU and is attained between 15 and 30 min after injection. Systematic studies by Hübener (1978) showed density increases of ca. 25 HU in the liver at approximately 60 min after contrast administration.

Hübener (1978) described only two applications for biliary contrast media in CT studies:

1. Demonstration of the extrahepatic biliary tract for identification of the hepatic duct, the common bile duct, and the papilla of Vater, especially for clarification of altered anatomic relations in the postoperative state.
2. Differentiation between healthy and diseased liver tissue, especially in focal nodular hyperplasia (FNH).

There have also been attempts at using contrast media which do not contain iodine and which possess a specific affinity for certain organs or lesions. Several authors have reported their initial experiences with new contrast media such as an iodinated fat emulsion which increases density in healthy tissue within the liver and the spleen but which is not taken up by hepatic and splenic tumors. There have also been experiments with contrast media containing solid material, elements with atomic numbers ranging between 1 and 83, and water-soluble iodinated iosefamatmeglumine.

To date dynamic CT studies have been performed with the same ionic and nonionic water-soluble contrast media containing iodine that are used in angiographic and urographic studies. The following characteristics of these compounds have led to their use for CT studies:

1. Iodine is the only chemical element with the following properties essential for contrast material: high contrast density, chemical characteristics which allow a wide variety of combinations with benzene molecules, and relatively low toxicity.
2. The symmetrically substituted triiodobenzene molecule demonstrates relatively strong iodine bonds as well as an extremely high proportion of iodine (approx. 91%).
3. The remaining three positions on the benzene ring are available for combinations with a number of side chains, which permits considerable variation in the physicochemical and biologic characteristics of the molecule.

4.2 Chemical Structure of Water-Soluble Contrast Media

Most ionic contrast media are based on amidotrizoate, a strong acid with a carboxyl group on the triiodobenzene ring and relatively water-soluble salts. The two side chains (–$NHCOCH_3$) increase water solubility and decrease protein binding. This results in good tolerance and exclusively renal excretion by means of glomerular filtration.

Metrizamide is a nonionic contrast agent derived from amidotrizoate. The solubility of this compouned does not result from ion bonds but rather from hydrophilic glucosamine joined to the molecule by an acid amine bond. This results in a low rate of local reactions. The hydrophilic characteristics of the molecule prevent intracellular penetration of the contrast medium.

4.3 Physical and Chemical Characteristics of Contrast Media

The physical and chemical characteristics of a contrast agent include solubility, viscosity, osmotic pressure, lipophilic or hydrophilic properties, electric charge, and protein binding.

Water solubility is a limiting factor in the manufacture of highly concentrated contrast media. Meglumine salts such as Angiografin are generally more soluble than sodium salts such as Urovison-sodium. Viscosity of contrast material, which is directly related to concentration and indirectly proportional to temperature, is decisive in determining the flow characteristics of contrast media in the blood. Contrast material is warmed to body temperature (37°C) in order to approximate the viscosity of blood. However, contrast media with the same iodine concentration and the same temperature may vary in viscosity independent of concentration. Viscosity is an important factor even at high injection rates and declines with increasing tangential forces which develop during injection.

Osmotic presure of contrast media determines one of the basic pharmacologic and toxicologic effects of the contrast medium. Osmotic pressure is proportional to the number of free particles such as molecules and ions per kilogram of water and is, unlike viscosity, related to concentration and – to a lesser extent – to temperature. However, contrast media with identical iodine concentrations may demonstrate widely different osmotic pressures. All contrast media used currently in radiology are hypertonic as compared with blood, though considerable effort has been expended on pharmaceutical research in the development of slightly hypertonic and isotonic contrast agents.

The lipophilic properties of a contrast medium are defined by its distribution between a lipophilic medium and a buffered aqueous solution at various pH values; this relation is termed the distribution coefficient. A contrast medium should have limited lipophilic characteristics, since the latter are associated with side effects. Lipophilic properties are reduced by electric charge, acid groups, and oxygen and nitrogen atoms in the side chains, while the presence of methyl groups increases the lipophilic characteristics of a contrast agent.

Water-soluble contrast media containing iodine are salts which are rendered more soluble by the addition of iodine-free bases, usually sodium or meglumine. The cations administered with the contrast medium dissociate from the contrast medium once in the blood. Knöfel et al. (1974) and Taenzer et al. (1981) stated that the free cations do not influence the pharmacokinetics of contrast media. Meglumine, like the anions in the contrast medium, is distributed primarily in the extracellular space and is eliminated by the kidneys. It has the following advantages over sodium salts: better solubility, less vascular irritation, fewer cardiovascular effects, and limited influence on the blood-brain barrier. Sodium salts possess some advantages over meglumine, such as lower viscosity, less histamine release, and more limited diuretic effects.

Intravenous administration of contrast media may result in hemodynamic effects which must be considered in radiologic studies of organ function. Schröder et al. (1981) described three phases in the hemodynamic effects resulting from intra-arterial administration of contrast media. The first phase is characterized by increased flow and pressure as well as by turbulence resulting from the kinetic energy contributed by the contrast medium. The second phase demonstrates reduced flow secondary to the high viscosity of the contrast medium. The third phase shows increased flow, which Schröder et al. (1981) attributed to the high osmolality of the contrast medium.

Increased flow is accompanied by a decrease in arterial blood pressure, caused by vasodilation secondary to the hyperosmolality of the contrast medium. Intravenous administration of contrast media in the pulmonary vascular bed results in increased pressure caused by a decreased flow in the capillary bed which is attributed to changes in the flow characteristics of the blood. In vivo and in vitro studies have shown that hyperosmolar contrast media cause aggregation of blood cells, especially of the red blood cells, with a consequent decrease in the flow characteristics of the blood, especially in the capillary bed. In addition, intravenous contrast administration may cause disorders of cardiac automaticity with changes in heart rate, especially bradycardia.

Contrast media may result in alterations in the venous endothelium, which can cause thrombosis.

4.4 Physiologic Aspects of Contrast Media Distribution

After intravenous administration contrast media are subject to the same distribution during the early phase as the blood itself.

Contrast media are transported exclusively in the plasma, which comprises approximately 55%–60% of the circulating blood volume. The corpuscular elements of the blood volume, termed hematocrit, make up approximately 41%–46% of the total volume and include the white and red blood cells which are transported in suspension in the blood plasma. Blood viscosity – the forces which develop between adjacent layers of blood – is related to hematocrit and averages 4.5 mPa in the healthy adult, as compared with 2.2 mPa for the plasma itself.

The total blood volume represents approximately 77 ± 7.7 ml/kg body weight or $\frac{1}{13}$ of body weight, which equals 5.4 liters in males, as compared with 4.5 liters or $\frac{1}{15}$ of body weight in females.

Albert (1971) determined that approximately 75% of total blood volume is found in the venous system and 15%–20% in the arterial vessels, with 7% of blood volume in the heart, 9% in the pulmonary circulation, and the remaining 84% in the blood vessels in the rest of the body. The capillary vessels have a comparatively small cross-sectional area and contain 16% of total blood volume.

The intravascular, interstitial, and intracellular spaces are the three large fluid compartments of the body. The interstitial fluid is involved in rapid exchange with the blood plasma as a result of the large surface area of the capillary walls. There is a concentration gradient for protein between the plasma and the interstitial fluid, because the capillary membrane is relatively impermeable for protein. Approximately 90% of plasma consists of water, and 6.58% of protein. A human being weighing 70 kg has the following volumes in the three major fluid compartments: 3.5 liters of blood plasma, 10 liters of interstitial fluid, and 30 liters of intracellular fluid.

The osmotic pressure of plasma – a measure of the total concentration of soluble materials – is 7.3 atm. Solutions with the same osmotic pressure as plasma are designated isotonic solutions. The resistance of the semipermeable cell membrane to the passage of many substances is so great that changes in osmotic pressure in the extracellular fluid may be followed by considerable transfers of water between the cell and the surrounding extracellular space. Low osmotic pressure in the extracellular space results in movement of water into the cell, with swelling of the latter and an increase in the volume of the intracellular compartment, which may ultimately result in destruction of the cell membrane. Hypertonic solutions in the extracellular space result in increased movement of water out of the cell.

Hemodynamic parameters play a major role in the distribution of contrast agents. The distribution of blood in the systemic circulation is determined by pressure gradients within the vascular bed. The pressure gradients overcome the resistance to flow maintained by the viscosity of the blood, the friction and inertia of the blood within the vascular system, and the peripheral vascular resistance.

According to the law of continuity, flow (volume per unit of time) is equal at all points whitin a system at a given time. In the human body the total cross-sectional area of all peripheral vessels is considerably larger than the cross-sectional area of the centrally located vessel. For this reason the rate of flow in the periphery is significantly lower and indirectly proportional to the total cross-sectional area of all vessels. The mean rate of flow in the aorta at rest is approximately 20 cm/s. In almost all parts of the circulatory system, inertia and friction at the vascular wall contribute to the development of adhesion and cohesion which result in lower flow rates near the vascular wall than in the middle of the vessel. Laminar flow demonstrates a parabolic flow profile, with the highest rate at the center and rates approaching zero at the periphery.

Exchange between the intravascular and interstitial spaces takes place in the capillaries, so the latter are the most important segment of the circulatory system in terms of function. Diffusion is the most important process in the exchange of fluid and other substances between the blood and the interstitial fluid. The high rate of exchange implies virtually continual mixing of plasma and the interstitial fluid. In addition to diffusion, filtration and reabsorption are involved in the exchange processes in the peripheral circulation.

Resistance within the organ correlates with transit time, from which the arteriovenous passage time – the interval between maximum concentration in the afferent artery and in the efferent vein – is calculated. These intervals have been established with conventional angiographic studies and range between 6 and 8 s for the brain (Wegener 1980), 8 and 12 s for the kidneys, 4 and 7 s for the lungs, and 10 and 15 s for the liver when calculated at the hepatic artery and 15 and 30 s when calculated at the superior mesenteric artery.

The vascular relations of the liver constitute a special case. Twenty-five percent of the blood flow of the liver is delivered by the hepatic artery and 75% by the portal vein. One of the major factors in blood distribution to the various organs is cardiac output, calculated as the product of stroke volume and heart rate, which ranges from 5 to 7 liters per minute at rest, with increases in response to demand primarily by means of increased heart rate. Cardiac output is related to body weight, surface area, and oxygen consumption. In order to calculate volumes of contrast media appropriate to cardiac output, a simplified formula – generally 1 ml/kg body weight – is used, although it should be considered that cardiac output declines with age.

Circulation time is a measure of the speed of blood flow and is defined as the time interval for flow between two points in the vascular bed. Since the cardiovascular system is highly complex, circulation time – which is related to age, as is cardiac output (Fig. 8a, b) – cannot be used as an index of blood flow (volume per units of time) in dynamic CT studies. There is a clear relation between circulation time and cardiac output, but Selzer et al. (1968) found that circulation time is of limited importance in the clinical situation. Heuck and Vanselow (1970) found that circulation time, flow rate, and blood volume were necessary for evaluation of the vascular system.

Circulation times vary from one organ to another, the coronary system having a circulation time of only 10 s. The kidneys and the brain also have shorter circulation times than the other major organs.

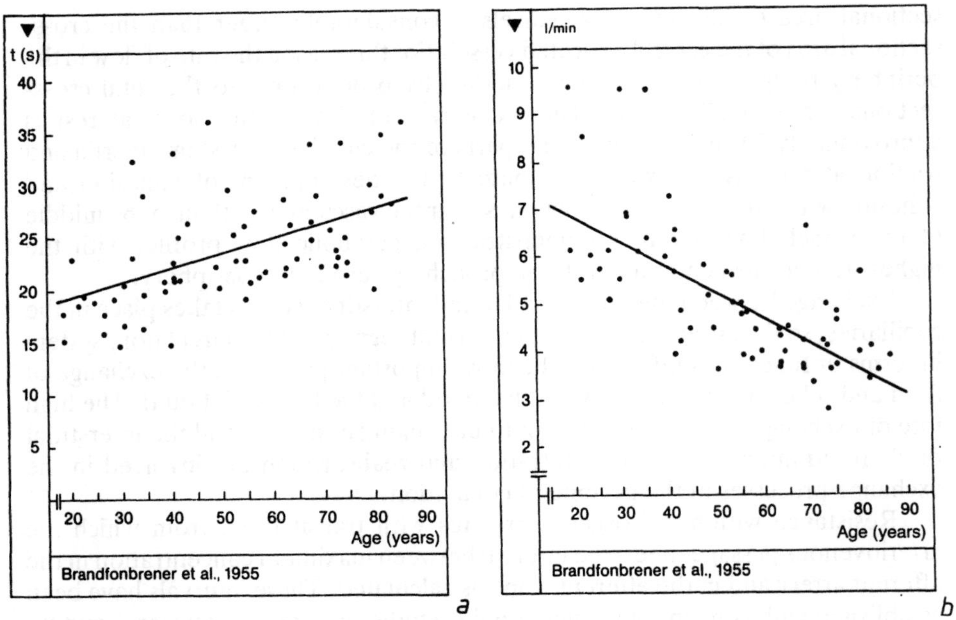

Fig. 8. a Relation of circulation time to age. Mean transit time from the antecubital vein to the brachial artery following injection of 5 mg T-1824. **b** Relation of cardiac output to age in 67 males without cardiovascular disease. (After Brandfonbrener et al. 1955)

4.5 Pharmacokinetics

Pharmacokinetics describe the time-dependent changes in concentration of contrast agents in the blood and tissues of individual organs, which are related to the chemical and physicochemical properties of contrast media described above. Hemodynamic factors are also significant.

A basic assumption in studying the pharmacokinetics of contrast media is that water-soluble contrast media do not interact with the organism. There is no evidence to date that strongly hydrophilic ionic or nonionic contrast media enter intact cells – with the exception of the hepatocytes – since contrast media are not transported across cell membranes. Meglumine does not penetrate the cell membrane, in contrast to sodium. Contrast media are mixed with the blood and transported to the periphery of the circulatory system, where they pass through the pores of the capillary endothelium into the interstitial space. Protein binding of water-soluble contrast media attains a maximum of only a few percent, and pharmacokinetic studies do not have to take metabolic processes into account.

Diffusion from the intravascular to the extravascular space depends primarily on the osmotic pressure of plasma, hydrostatic pressure, and the permeability of the capillary wall. The concentrations of dissolved substances, proteins, and contrast media in the plasma influence the osmotic pressure of circulating blood,

Fig. 9a, b. Schematic illustration of contrast enhancement in the intravascular and interstitial spaces. **a** In the brain: *left,* immediately after bolus injection; *right,* after several circulatory cycles. **b** In the body: *left,* immediately after bolus injection; *right,* after several circulatory cycles

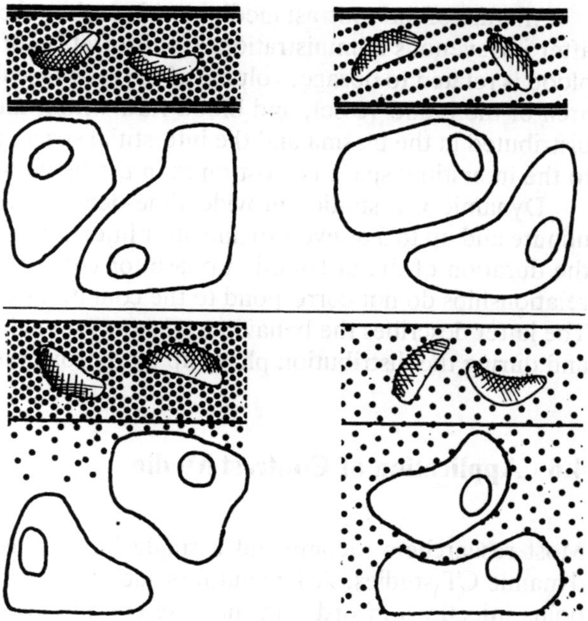

which, in turn, influences the transfer of substances to the semipermeable membrane. Changes in plasma osmolality also result in alterations in the size and shape of red blood cells, with a direct influence on the flow characteristics of the blood. Excretion of contrast media by glomerular filtration takes place simultaneously with the processes described above, and evaluation of dynamic CT studies must take this factor into account, paying special attention to the glomerular filtration rate. Dynamic CT studies measure changes in density within the first minutes after contrast application, and renal excretion can be disregarded to a certain extent, since the half-lives of various contrast media range from 80 to 120 min.

The particular conditions of brain tissue deserve special attention. Under normal conditions, contrast media do not cross the blood-brain barrier to enter the small interstitial space of the brain. An increase in contrast within the brain is due solely to the presence of contrast medium within the blood vessels (Fig. 9a). Disruption of the blood-brain barrier allows passage of contrast medium from the intravascular to the interstitial space. In other organs the interstitial space is considerably larger, comprising 10%–25% of the fluid volume of the organ.

After intravenous administration, contrast medium is distributed throughout the plasma space, and most of the contrast agent passes into the interstitial space after the first passage through the capillary bed (Fig. 9b). Approximately 15% of the contrast medium remains in the interstitial space of the pulmonary vascular bed before the contrast material reaches the arterial vessels.

Increased density in the blood vessels is solely related to the concentration of contrast medium in the blood, while density increases in tissues also depend on regional blood flow, vascular perfusion, and interstitial distribution of the contrast medium.

Mixture of the contrast medium with the blood occurs rapidly, within 15–30 s after intravenous administration. Concentration of the contrast material in the blood is related to dosage, volume of the intravascular space, the cross-sectional area of the blood vessel, and blood flow within the vessel. Contrast media are distributed in the plasma and the interstitial space, and passage from the plasma to the interstitial space is most rapid in the tissue with the greatest blood flow.

Dynamic CT studies provide time-density measurements within the first minute and up to 5 or even 10 min after injection. These periods are shorter than the duration of the distribution phase for contrast media, and the time-density relationships do not correspond to the conditions of a two-compartment model. The latter describes the behaviour of contrast media after mixing with the blood and during the distribution phase up to approximately 120 min after injection.

4.6 Application of Contrast Media

Most researchers recommend a single bolus injection of contrast material in dynamic CT studies. A few authors such as Rossi et al. (1981) prefer multiple bolus injections in order to increase contrast enhancement in the vessels and organs.

Wegener (1980a) differentiated between targeted and controlled bolus injection. The former is preferable when strong contrast over a short period is desired. This is particularly relevant to contrast enhancement in blood vessels and organs. Hacker and Becker (1977) were the first to report time-related angiographic studies with CT and recommended targeted bolus injection in order to obtain the best possible contrast enhancement in vessels and organs with CT systems characterized by short scan times and long scan intervals. CT studies are made after the bolus of contrast medium reaches the target organ, in order to record the greatest possible contrast enhancement within the organ.

Controlled bolus injection is designed to achieve contrast enhancement in the blood vessels and heart for a period of 3–5 min. This form of bolus injection is primarily used in cardio-CT studies, in order to achieve maximum contrast delineation of the ventricle against the septum and the ventricular walls. Reduced bolus injection involves application of 5–10 ml of contrast medium, 10–15 min before a CT examination, in order to achieve contrast enhancement of the urinary bladder.

Continuous administration of a contrast agent is employed in order to achieve high contrast over a longer period of time (3–15 min, for example) especially for demonstration of large vascular distributions (Fig. 10).

The rate of contrast administration is determined by the rate of increase and maintenance of contrast enhancement, since contrast agents pass from the blood vessels into the interstitial space and are eliminated by the kidneys during administration of the contrast medium. For this reason a combination of bolus injection and infusion may be employed, e.g., for demonstration of the mediastinum. Bolus administration of 1 ml of contrast medium per kilogram of body weight is followed by a continuous infusion in order to maintain contrast

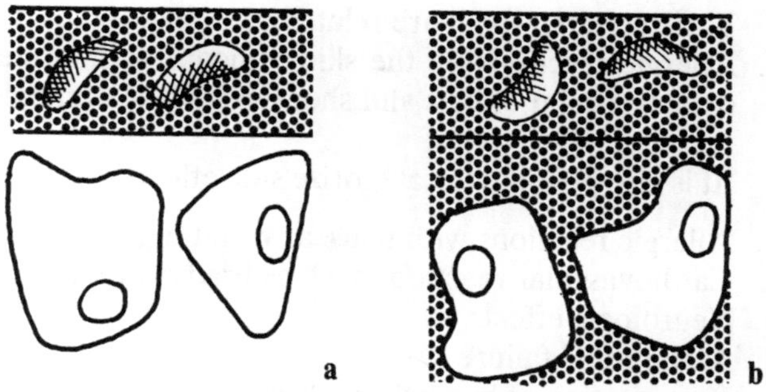

Fig. 10a, b. Schematic illustration of contrast enhancement: **a** following bolus injection; **b** with continuous intravenous infusion

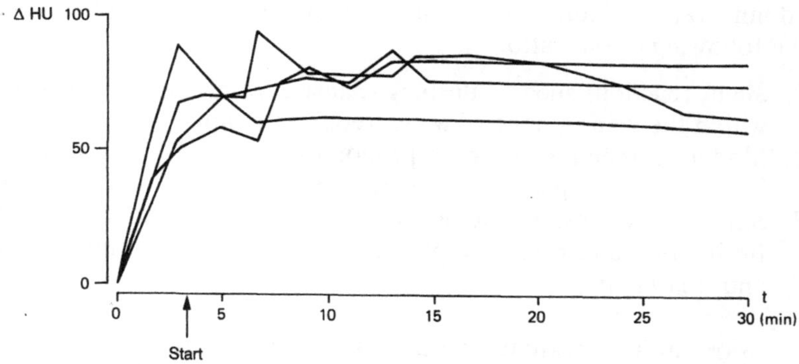

Fig. 11. Contrast enhancement in the thoracic aorta with continuous infusion. Initial rapid infusion over 7 min followed by reducion in flow rate to 1.5 g I/min, in order to maintain contrast enhancement at 60–80 HU over a prolonged period

enhancement. The rate of infusion is adjusted to maintain a desired concentration in the blood. Total dosages of iodine may attain 60–80 g with this technique (Fig. 11).

4.7 Side effects

In 1980 Shehadi and Toniolo published an international multicenter study involving 300000 patients who had undergone various studies with contrast media and reported a complication rate of 4.73%. These results are lower than those found by Ansell (8.5%) in 1970 and Witten et al. (7%) in 1973.

It is possible to categorize side effects of contrast media in several ways. Lange et al. (1979) differentiated between generalized toxic reactions and local reactions. Others have classified side effects according to their causes:

1. Toxic effects, which are related to dosage
2. Allergic reactions on the skin, mucous membranes, and airways, including cardiovascular effects and shock, which are generally unrelated to dosage.

It is also possible to categorize side effects according to symptoms and signs:

1. Allergic reactions with nausea, vomiting, urticaria, airway obstruction, etc.
2. Cardiovascular reactions such as bradycardia, tachycardia, and hypotension
3. Neurologic effects
4. Acute renal failure
5. Precipitation of hyperthyroidism

In clinical practice side effects are usually characterized according to their severity, in order to develop means of treating complications related to the administration of contrast material. Frommhold and Hausdörfer (1976) provided the following classification:

1. Slight reactions such as flushing, nausea, vomiting, mild urticaria, and pain within the veins – none of which require therapy
2. Moderate reactions such as pronounced urticaria, edema of the face and larynx, bronchospasm, and severe hypotension – all of which require therapy
3. Severe reactions, including collapse, protracted hypotension, ventricular fibrillation, and renal complications, which require immediate intervention and treatment

Most authors attribute the side effects of contrast media to an idiosyncratic reaction to the whole molecule rather than to the iodine alone. Ring (1979) postulated a complex interaction of a number of systems involving histamine release from basophilic granulocytes and mast cells coupled with complement activation. In vitro studies have also demonstrated inhibition of the coagulation process. The symptoms and signs of reactions to contrast media have also implicated an immune response as a factor, and antibodies have been demonstrated in patients suffering severe reactions to contrast media. However, Schatz et al. (1975) demonstrated that repeated reactions to contrast media were found in only 16% of patients who had suffered an initial episode, which casts doubt on the hypothesis of an allergic reaction as the cause.

The "anxiety hypothesis" proposed by Lalli and Greenstreet (1981) has claimed considerable interest in the past few years. Lalli suggested that activity in the central nervous system originating in the frontal lobes and the hypothalamus may initiate reactions which are capable of causing pulmonary edema, cardiac arrest, coagulation disorders, nausea, and skin eruptions (Fig. 12).

Renal damage up to and including acute renal failure is one of the most serious complications attributed to the administration of contrast media. The risk is particularly high in cases of dehydration and in patients with type I diabetes mellitus. Renal damage takes the form of oliguria and an increase in serum creatinine.

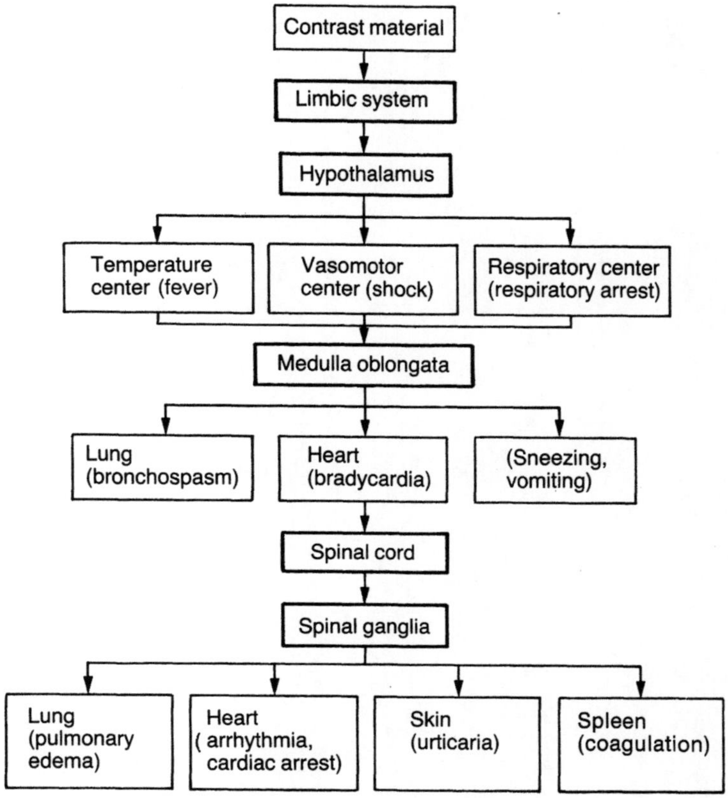

Fig. 12. Possible interactions between contrast material and the central nervous system (after Lalli)

5 Bolus Geometry and Dynamics: Contrast Studies with Intravenous Contrast Media

Dynamic CT studies develop time-density measurements in order to demonstrate the distribution of contrast media in blood vessels and organs over time.

Relatively long scan times up to 5 s and scan intervals up to 4 s do not permit accurate descriptions of bolus geometry and contrast dynamics with this method.

As is the case with angiodensitometric methods in conventional angiography, rapid sequences of studies in the chronogram permit analysis of temporal changes in contrast density after bolus injection of contrast material in large vessels. The method is similar to indicator dilution studies and provides curves representing "dilution" of contrast media as a noninvasive technique for determining temporal changes in iodine concentration within the vessels.

Between 10 and 20 s after bolus injection of contrast material there is a steep increase in density over the aorta during the first passage of the contrast agent, followed by a rapid, somewhat less steep decline in density to a first minimum density value. In most cases there is a second lower peak caused by recirculation of the contrast material. Mean density curves describe a rapid decrease in density in the aorta within the first minute independent of the rate of injection and the dose of contrast material (Fig. 13). Complete mixing of a contrast agent with the

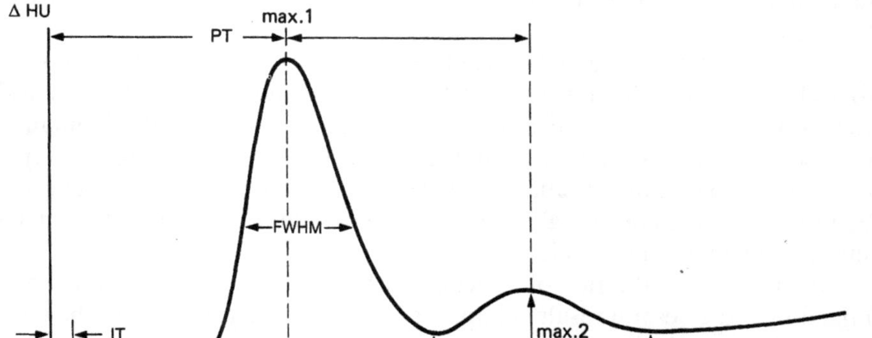

Fig. 13. Schematic illustration of density values corresponding to time-density measurements in serial CT studies and chronograms. Density values in the aorta during two circulatory cycles following intravenous administration of a contrast agent. *IT*, injection time; *AT*, arrival time; *PT*, peak time; *FWHM*, full width half maximum; *max. 1*, first peak; *max. 2*, second peak; *min. 1*, first density minimum after first peak

blood has usually been completed by this point, which corresponds to approximately four complete circulatory cycles. Experiments in laboratory animals have shown that administration of a highly concentrated solution of contrast medium containing 300 mg iodine per milliliter is so thoroughly diluted during the first circulatory cycle that the maximum concentration of iodine at the time of maximum contrast enhancement is only 10% of the original iodine concentration in the solution. Mixture of contrast medium with the blood is accompanied by simultaneous diffusion into the interstitial space and excretion by glomerular filtration, which contributes to a further decrease in contrast density in the blood. Plasma half-life in the interval between 52 and 300 s after injection is found at approximately 3 min on a virtually exponential curve which corresponds to the known half-life for distribution in classic pharmacokinetic studies of contrast media. Half-times for renal excretion are considerably longer – generally between 80 and 120 min in humans – and have little influence on distribution of contrast medium in the first few seconds after injection.

Dosage recommendations for contrast media are related to body weight, generally 1 ml/kg body weight, in order to attain adequate contrast enhancement, especially in soft tissue organs. This results in various volumes of contrast material for patients with different weights, which implies that duration of injection varies at a constant flow rate (8 ml/s, for example) in patients with different weights.

Peak attenuation is a function of the duration of injection, which can be controlled by varying the volume of contrast medium or the rate of injection. Our studies have shown that heart rate also has an influence on peak attenuation values, as Schad et al. (1981) have also reported. As a result, volume of contrast medium, rate of injection, and heart rate must be considered in estimating the point in time at which maximum attenuation is to be attained.

Even when the relations described above are considered, there may be individual unforeseeable deviations from the expected peak of contrast enhancement. The lung is usually the source of these alterations as a result of its reservoir function.

The lung may also serve as a volume buffer for the bolus of contrast medium to such an extent that an increase in the flow rate above 8 ml/s results in a slight reduction in the interval until peak attenuation is achieved. A significant increase in maximum contrast enhancement is not attainable, but the increased injection rates raise pressure in the cubital vein to such an extent that contrast material may be forced into the peripheral veins. This phenomenon is also observed in digital subtraction angiography (Fig. 14a).

An increase in the rate of injection with constant volume and reduced total injection time does not result in improved contrast in organs such as the liver and spleen. Increased rate of injection does shorten the interval until peak attenuation, but this result is not statistically significant. Rate of injection does not significantly affect the level and duration of maximum contrast enhancement in soft tissue structures (Fig. 14b).

Administration of a bolus of physiologic saline solution does not change bolus geometry and dynamics in the aorta, and this maneuver is unnecessary in dynamic CT studies and digital subtraction angiography.

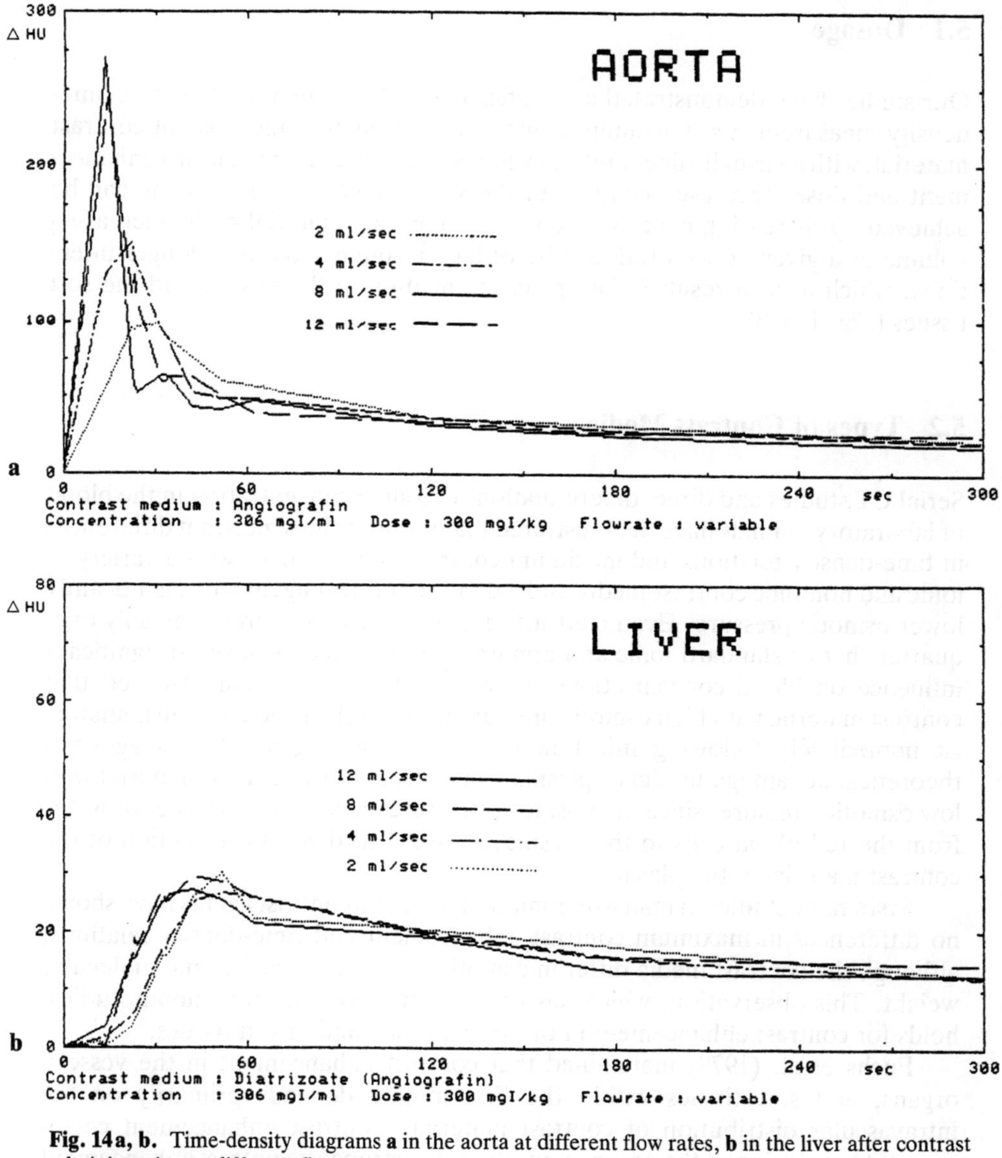

Fig. 14a, b. Time-density diagrams **a** in the aorta at different flow rates, **b** in the liver after contrast administration at different flow rates

The first scan in the series should be made between 11 and 16 s after the beginning of injection in order to establish the peak of contrast enhancement in the aorta.

Exact timing is probably not necessary, since passage of the contrast medium through the heart and lungs tends to spread the bolus. Scan times of approximately 5 s make it likely that the bolus of contrast material will be detected in the CT scan.

5.1 Dosage

Our studies have demonstrated a statistically significant relation between time-density measurements, maximum contrast enhancement, and dose of contrast material, with a virtually linear relationship between maximum contrast enhancement and dose. Increased contrast in the vascular bed and soft tissue can be achieved by increasing concentration of the contrast material or by increasing volume at a given concentration. Use of larger volumes requires longer injections, which in turn result in late peak attenuation in the vessels and the soft tissues (Fig. 15a, b).

5.2 Types of Contrast Media

Serial CT studies and direct determinations of iodine concentration in the blood of laboratory animals have demonstrated that there are no significant differences in time-density relations and maximum contrast enhancement with a variety of ionic and nonionic contrast media and a dimeric contrast agent with significantly lower osmotic pressure. Even contrast media with osmotic pressures only one-quarter that of standard ionic and nonionic contrast agents have no significant influence on blood concentrations. However, it has been demonstrated that contrast material with high osmotic pressure causes a clear reduction in hematocrit immediately following injection of the contrast agent. This suggests a theoretical advantage in higher plasma concentrations of contrast material with low osmotic pressure, since high osmotic pressure causes a net transfer of water from the red blood cells to the plasma, resulting in theoretical dilution of the contrast material in the plasma.

Systematic studies in man with ionic and nonionic contrast agents have shown no differences in maximum contrast enhancement and time-density relations, although the contrast media differ in osmotic pressure, viscosity, and molecular weight. This observation, which has been verified with chronographic studies, holds for contrast enhancement in the vascular bed and in soft tissues.

Fuchs et al. (1979) maintained that contrast enhancement in the vessels, organs, and soft tissues within the first minute depends primarily on the intravascular distribution of contrast material. Contrast enhancement corresponds to perfusion of the organ in question; the strongest contrast enhancement is found in organs with the greatest blood flow. Therefore contrast material in the vascular bed is of primary importance for dynamic CT studies, since the contrast enhancement within the first minute is related to dilution and distribution of contrast material in the blood vessels, although there may be significant passage of contrast material from the vessels to the interstitial space in highly vascular organs. This phenomenon may be observed during the passage of a contrast agent through the lungs. Distribution of contrast material between the vascular bed and the interstitial space is complete after approximately 60 s; the subsequent decline in density values within soft tissue structures is determined by the amount of contrast medium in the interstitial space of these organs.

a

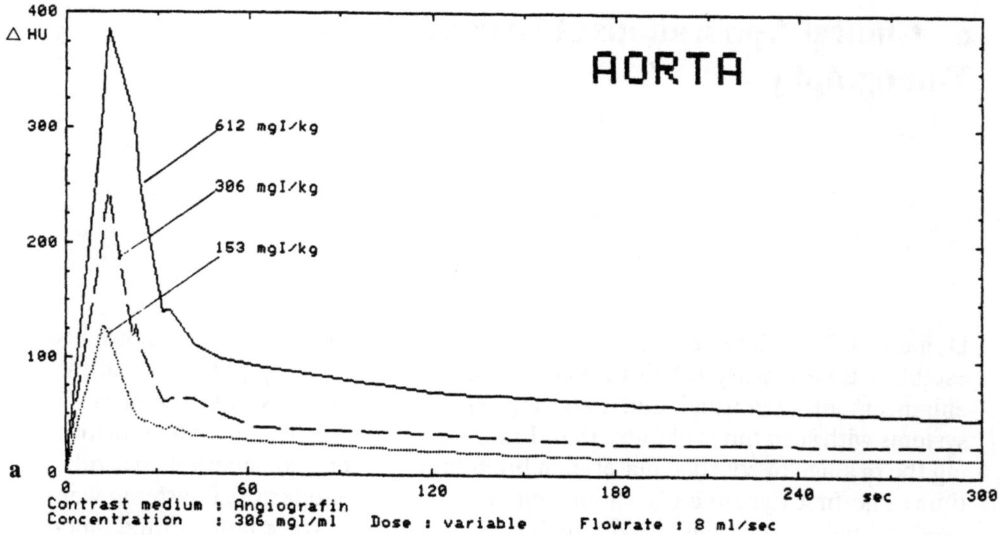

b

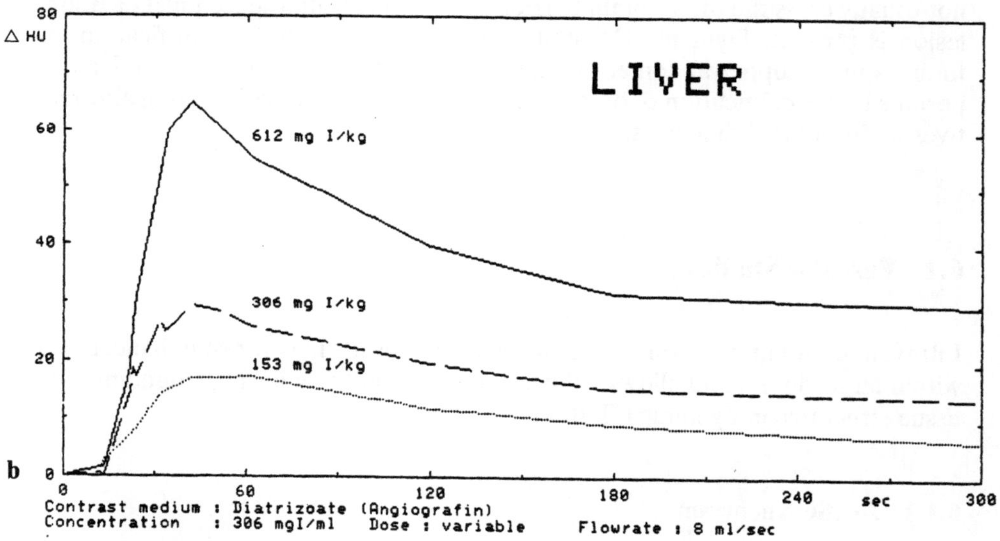

Fig. 15. **a** Time-density curves in the aorta as a function of volume of the contrast agent. **b** Time-density diagrams in the liver with various volumes of contrast agent

6 Clinical Applications of Dynamic Computed Tomography

Dynamic CT studies can be made for any organ or tissue in the body, in order to establish time-density relations which demonstrate the early phase of contrast enhancement in normal and pathologically altered tissues. First generation systems with scan times of more than 1 min per slice were capable of demonstrating the passage of contrast material in brain tumors over a considerable period of time. The first dynamic CT studies made with more modern CT systems were used to analyse regional blood circulation in the brain, since contrast media do not usually cross the blood-brain barrier into the interstitial space unless a brain lesion is present. Dynamic CT studies are used primarily for clarification of findings in the upper abdomen, where demonstration of differences in density permits better delineation of organic lesions and improved definition of alternatives in differential diagnosis.

6.1 Vascular Studies

Intravenous administration of contrast material results in contrast enhancement within large vessels and allows delineation of the latter against surrounding soft tissue structures in dynamic CT studies.

6.1.1 Aortic Aneurysm

Until several years ago, clinical suspicion of a thoracic or abdominal aneurysm required angiographic studies. A palpable abdominal aneurysm can often be demonstrated by means of diagnostic ultrasound, but the presence of gas in the intestines leads to misinterpretation in many cases. In addition, the results are sometimes not reproducible when studies are performed by inexperienced personnel.

CT studies allow demonstration of aneurysms and intravascular thrombi without the presence of motion artifacts. Modern systems are capable of demonstrating dissection and involvement of branching vessels. CT is a safe and noninvasive method which provides complete documentation of the location and extent of an aortic aneurysm with demonstration of aortic rupture and hemorrhage, which is of particular importance in planning surgical strategy (Fig. 16).

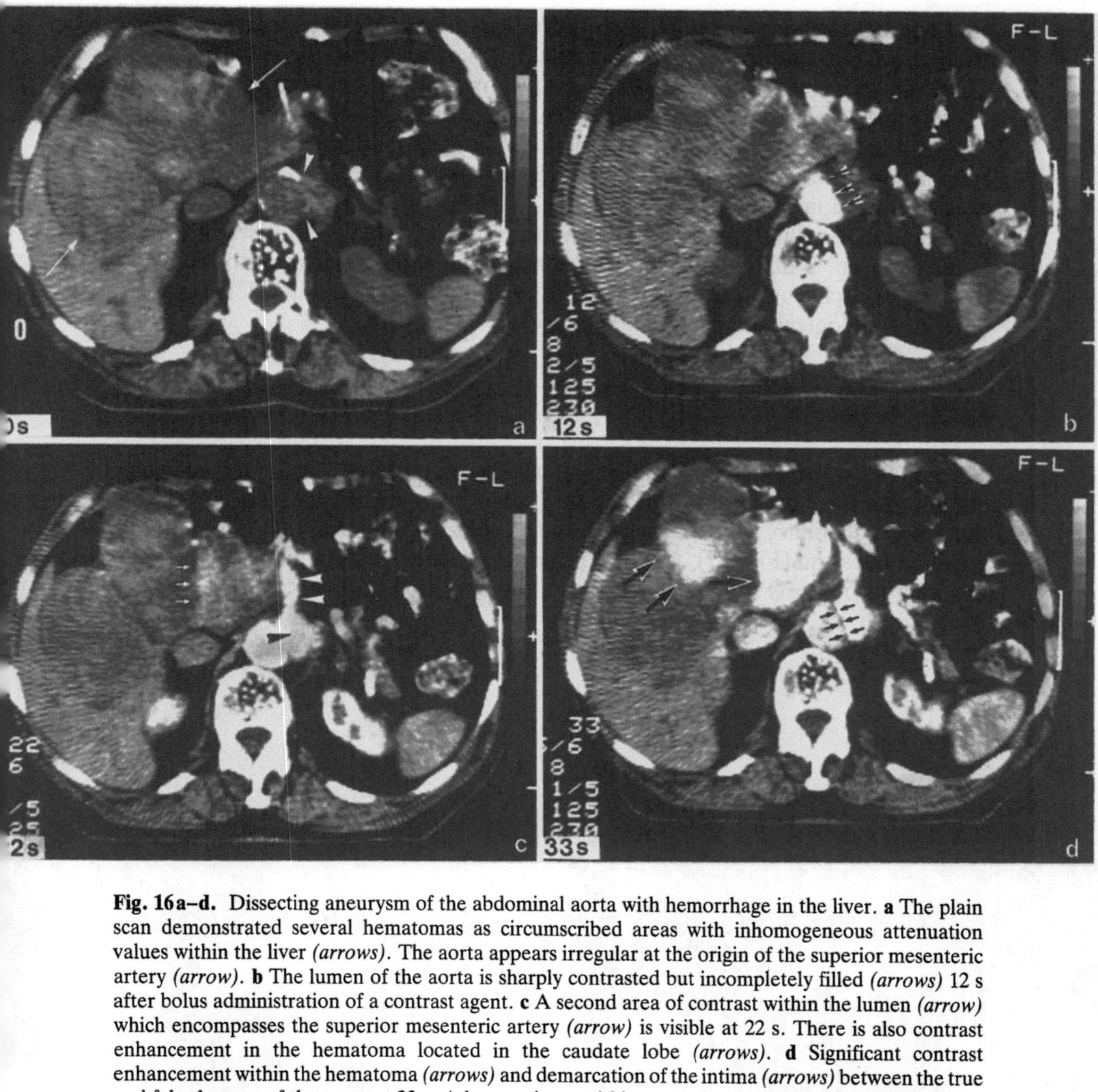

Fig. 16a–d. Dissecting aneurysm of the abdominal aorta with hemorrhage in the liver. **a** The plain scan demonstrated several hematomas as circumscribed areas with inhomogeneous attenuation values within the liver *(arrows)*. The aorta appears irregular at the origin of the superior mesenteric artery *(arrow)*. **b** The lumen of the aorta is sharply contrasted but incompletely filled *(arrows)* 12 s after bolus administration of a contrast agent. **c** A second area of contrast within the lumen *(arrow)* which encompasses the superior mesenteric artery *(arrow)* is visible at 22 s. There is also contrast enhancement in the hematoma located in the caudate lobe *(arrows)*. **d** Significant contrast enhancement within the hematoma *(arrows)* and demarcation of the intima *(arrows)* between the true and false lumens of the aorta at 33 s. A hemangioma within a vertebra is also visible in this slice

Dissection of the aorta requires rapid diagnosis. Conventional angiography has proved its worth in this situation. However, angiography entails certain risks, especially in older patients with renal and cardiovascular disorders. A safe, rapid, and noninvasive method such as CT provides the same diagnostic information at lower risk.

When dissection of the aorta or hemorrhage is suspected, a series of CT pictures (six or seven per minute) is made at the site of the suspected dissection following bolus injection of 1 ml (containing 300 mg iodine) of contrast material per kilogram of body weight. This is followed by studies made with an intravenous infusion of contrast material. If the aneurysm extends for 6 cm or less, the additional study with continous infusion of contrast medium is unnecessary.

In some cases serial CT studies are made after infusion when the first series of studies has failed to demonstrate the false lumen, and the strong contrast enhancement available with bolus injection and serial CT studies is required for exact localization of the lesion.

Serial CT studies also allow evaluation of renal perfusion in cases in which renal function is affected by involvement of the renal arteries with subtotal stenosis or occlusion in the aneurysm. In this situation CT studies demonstrate both morphological and functional changes.

6.1.2 Thrombosis

Thrombosis appears as a filling defect at the moment of maximum contrast enhancement following bolus injection of contrast material. Total occlusion of the vessel secondary to thrombosis prevents contrast enhancement in the blood vessel in question (Fig. 17). Collateral circulation may be demonstrated in cases in which thrombosis has persisted over a longer period of time.

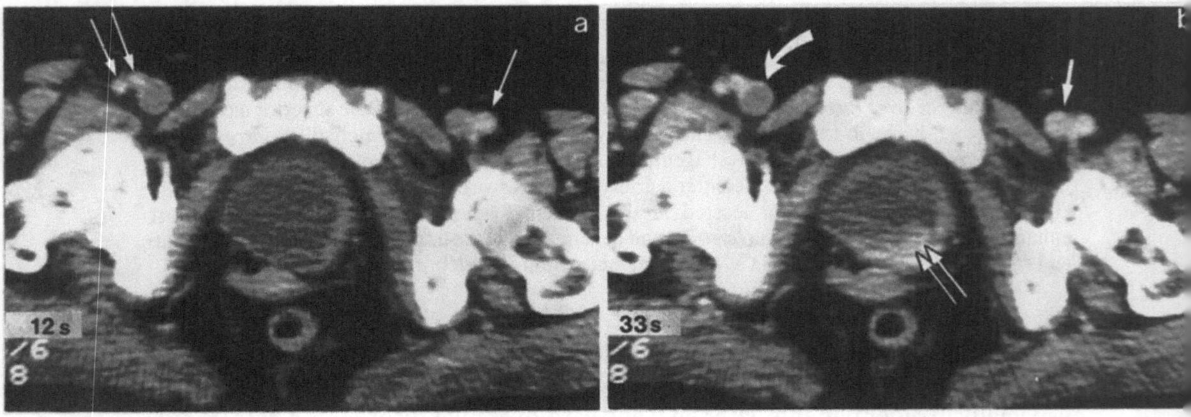

Fig. 17a, b. Thrombosis of the right femoral vein. **a** Contrast enhancement of the deep femoral and superficial femoral arteries *(arrows)* on the right and of the left common femoral artery *(arrow)* at 12 s. The right femoral vein is dilated. **b** Homogeneous contrast enhancement in the left femoral vein *(arrow)* at 33 s. The lumen of the right femoral vein *(arrow)* remains hypodense due to thrombosis. A hypervascular carcinoma, located in the posterior wall of the urinary bladder *(arrows)*, is also visible in this slice

6.2 Heart

CT is currently used primarily for the demonstration of intracavitary space-occupying lesions.

Experimental and comparative clinical studies are now being performed in order to evaluate the role of CT in demonstration of aortocoronary bypass grafts and in the diagnosis of coronary heart disease.

Contrast media aid in delineation of the ventricles and coronary vessels, since exact definition of the ventricle walls and the septum is not possible in plain scans. Demonstration of the intravascular space may be achieved in four ways:

1. Repeated administration of 10–20 ml of contrast material for each scan, with a total of 100–150 ml of contrast medium.
2. Initial contrast studies with 90 ml followed by repeated bolus injection of 10–20 ml to a total of 200–250 ml of contrast material.
3. Rapid intravenous infusion of 200 ml of contrast material. This offers the advantage of homogeneous contrast enhancement over a period of 10–15 min.
4. Bolus injection of 25–30 ml of contrast medium by means of an injection pump followed by rapid series of CT scans (six or seven scans per minute) in function studies, especially for demonstration of aortocoronary bypass grafts.

Most studies involve demonstration of morphological changes in different planes and functional conditions, and a large dose of a highly concentrated contrast agent such as Urografin 76% is necessary because of the long duration of the study.

6.2.1 Myocardial Infarction

Contrast studies in laboratory animals have demonstrated a delay in contrast enhancement in areas of acute myocardial infarction. Direct measurements of iodine concentration made with fluorescence methods have demonstrated delays in the accumulation of iodine in infarcted tissue with significantly higher values than in surrounding tissue at 10 min. The greatest differences between infarcted tissue and normal myocardium are measured at 150–180 min. Although the exact mechanism determining the distribution of contrast medium within infarcted myocardial tissue has not as yet been elucidated, delayed wash-out of contrast medium secondary to disordered perfusion is under discussion as a possible explanation.

Studies in laboratory animals and in man have produced similar results. The zone of infarction is hypodense immediately after administration of contrast material as a result of reduced perfusion in this area. At 10 min the area of infarction demonstrates higher density than surrounding tissue. Thinning of the myocardium has been demonstrated even in very small infarctions. In vitro studies have shown a linear correlation between the volume of infarcted tissue determined by CT studies and the actual extent of myocardial infarction.

Calculated values for infarction averaged up to 27% less than the actual values. The reason for this discrepancy might be the partial volume effect, since healthy tissue at the margins of the infarcted area may be included in an 8-mm slice. Another source of error may lie in the fact that cross-sectional slices are not always made at exactly 90° to the long axis of the heart. Modern scanners with scanning times longer than 1 s are still too limited for use in routine diagnosis of myocardial infarction.

Disorders of regional wall motion can be demonstrated with ECG-triggered cardio-CT studies (Fig. 18). However, the method is complicated and radiation exposure rather high, so the procedure is limited to two slices. Disorders of regional wall motion in the anterior region may be demonstrated in systole and diastole, which provides the possibility for calculating ejection fractions. Lackner et al. (1982) and Rienmüller et al. (1982) proved that CT is suitable for calculating ejection fractions on the basis of calculated endsystolic and enddiastolic volumes in different planes. Areas of past infarction present as low density zones which do not enhance at 10 min due to myocardial scarring, which differentiates these areas from acute infarction with increased contrast uptake at 10 min.

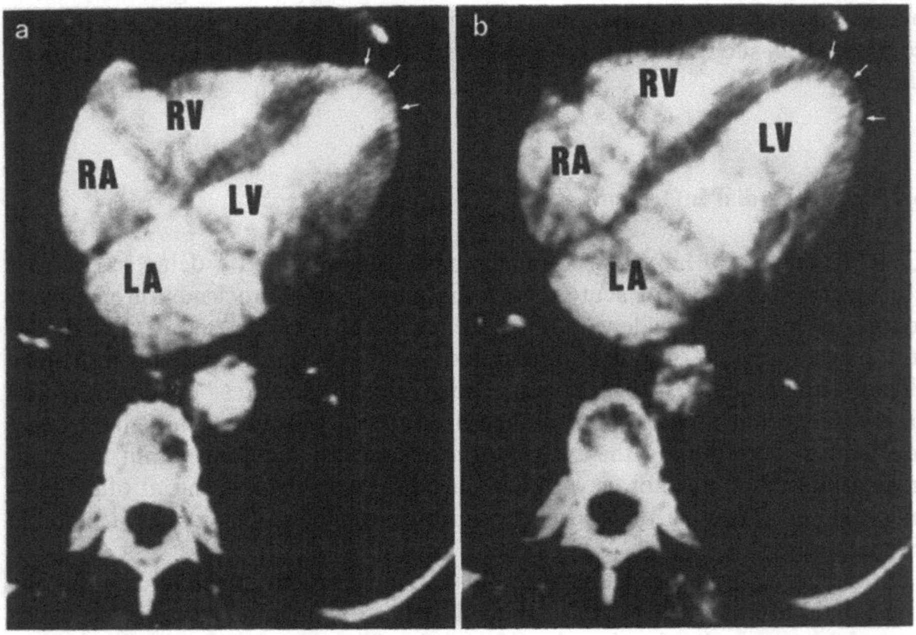

Fig. 18a, b. ECG-triggered CT study in a patient with anterior myocardial infarction. **a** Systole: the apical region of the left ventricle is thin and akinetic *(arrows)*, while the septum and lateral walls demonstrate normal contraction. Absence of contraction in the apical region results in protrusion of this segment. **b** Diastole: Loss of myocardial tissue is not apparent in this phase. *RV*, right ventricle; *LV* left ventricle; *LA*, left atrium; *RA*, right atrium

6.2.2 Ventricular Aneurysm

Ventricular aneurysm secondary to myocardial infarction is an indication for CT studies. The majority of aneurysms develop in the apex and the anterior wall; inferior aneurysms are much less common. Aneurysms are composed primarily of scar tissue but may contain viable myocardium.

Demonstration of aneurysms in the anterior and lateral regions of the left ventricle is usually successful, but the results are less favorable in inferior aneurysms. CT demonstrates protrusion and thinning of the ventricular wall. There is positive contrast enhancement in the aneurysm if circulation is sufficient, while scar tissue is demonstrated as a filling defect. Calcification within the ventricular wall in older aneurysms is easily demonstrated due to its high density values (Fig. 19).

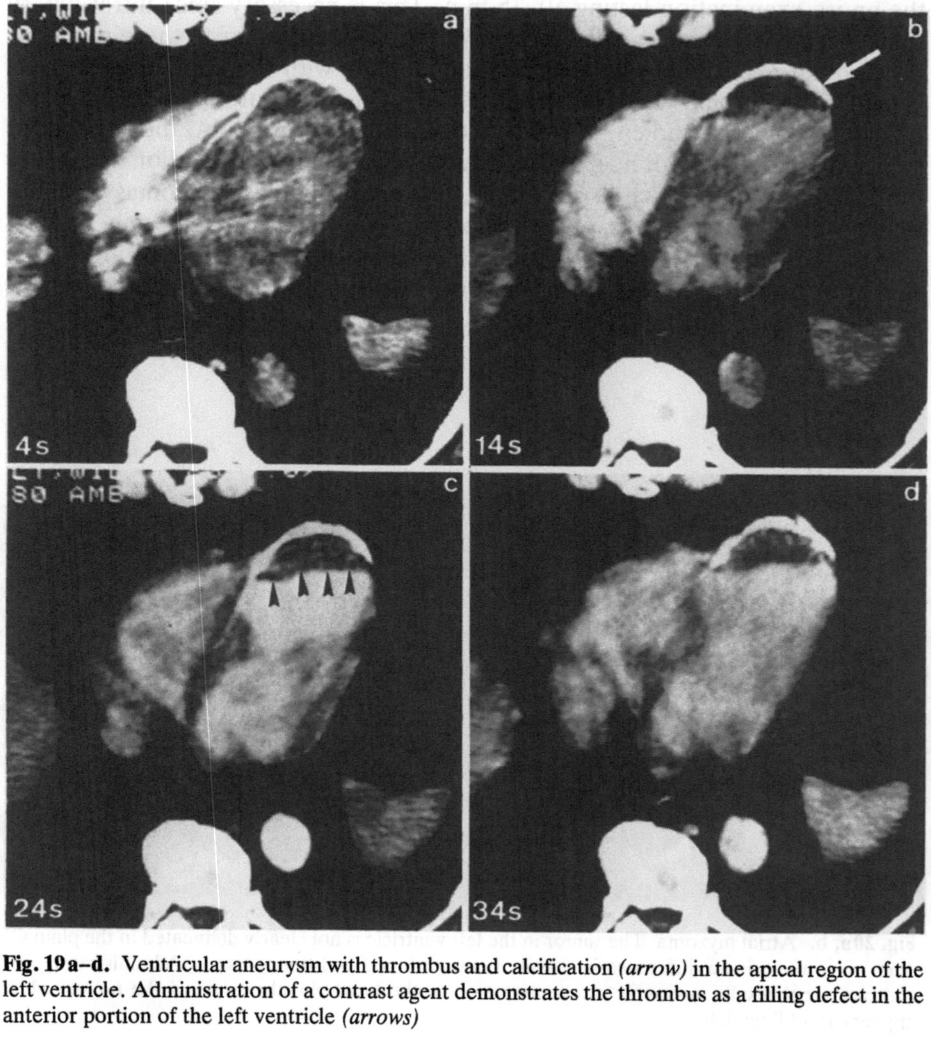

Fig. 19 a–d. Ventricular aneurysm with thrombus and calcification *(arrow)* in the apical region of the left ventricle. Administration of a contrast agent demonstrates the thrombus as a filling defect in the anterior portion of the left ventricle *(arrows)*

ECG-triggered cardio-CT studies are helpful in evaluation of regional wall motion in cases of aneurysm. Accurate delineation of the aneurysm is usually possible, especially in systole, since failure of this segment to contract makes protrusion of the ventricular wall in this area even more evident.

6.2.3 Intracavitary Space-Occupying Lesions: Thrombi and Tumors

Thrombi often develop in the left ventricle or the left atrium following myocardial infarction. Godwin et al. (1981) found thrombi in 20%–60% of cases at autopsy in myocardial infarction.

Adequate contrast enhancement is a prerequisite for diagnosis of an intracavitary space-occupying structure. This is achieved by means of continuous rapid infusion of highly concentrated contrast material (Urografin 76%) during the entire examination lasting 10–15 min. This is necessary since intracavitary space-occupying lesions generally have density values similar to those of blood. As in other CT studies, the examination is made with the patient holding his breath. The thrombi and other space-occupying structures appear as filling defects in contrast studies. Thrombi are classified according to their shapes as spherical, mural, or pedunculated structures (Fig. 19). Differentiation from other intracavitary tumors such as myxomas, fibromas, lipomas, angiomas, rhabdomyomas, and sarcomas is often impossible. Low density values in lipomas (– 80– – 100 HU) and cysts (0–20 HU) are characteristic and allow differentiation from other space-occupying lesions. History and other findings provide additional diagnostic help (Fig. 20).

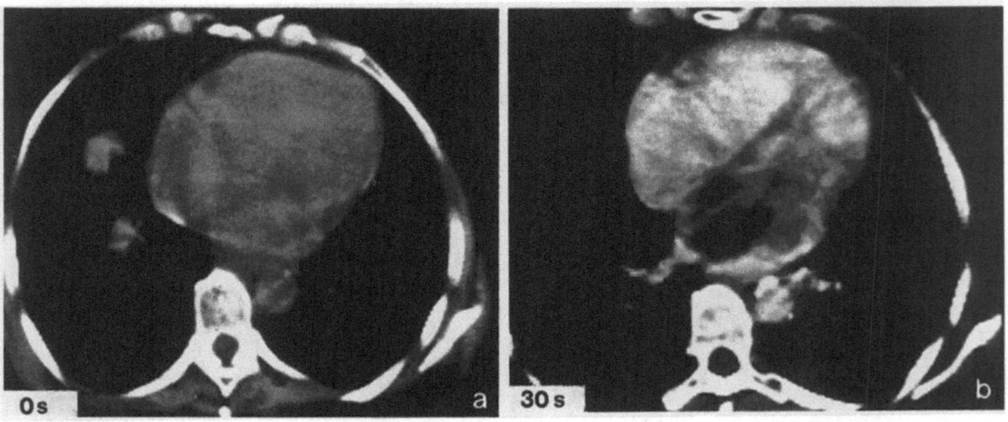

Fig. 20a, b. Atrial myxoma. The tumor in the left ventricle is not clearly delineated in the plain CT scan, since there is no difference in density between blood and tumor tissue. Administration of a contrast agent results in complete demonstration of the heart chambers and of the tumor, which appears as a filling defect

6.2.4 Aortocoronary Bypass Grafts

CT provides an opportunity to test the patency of bypass grafts. The bypass may be demonstrated in plain scans in some cases, though these studies do not permit conclusions on the function of the graft. Clips implanted at operation are a source of artifacts.

Intravenous administration of contrast material is a prerequisite for demonstration of a bypass graft. Studies are generally most successful when the catheter is located 1–2 cm from the metal clip and slightly below the bypass itself.

Two different procedures may be employed:

1. Administration of 50 ml of a highly concentrated contrast medium for initial studies, followed by additional injections of approximately 20 ml for each slice in the series. This technique allows demonstration of the entire heart and the bypass grafts in each slice, with consistently high contrast and clear delineation of the grafts from adjacent vessels, fat and myocardium.
2. Administration of a bolus of 25–30 ml of contrast medium, followed by dynamic CT studies in a preselected slice immediately below the origin of the

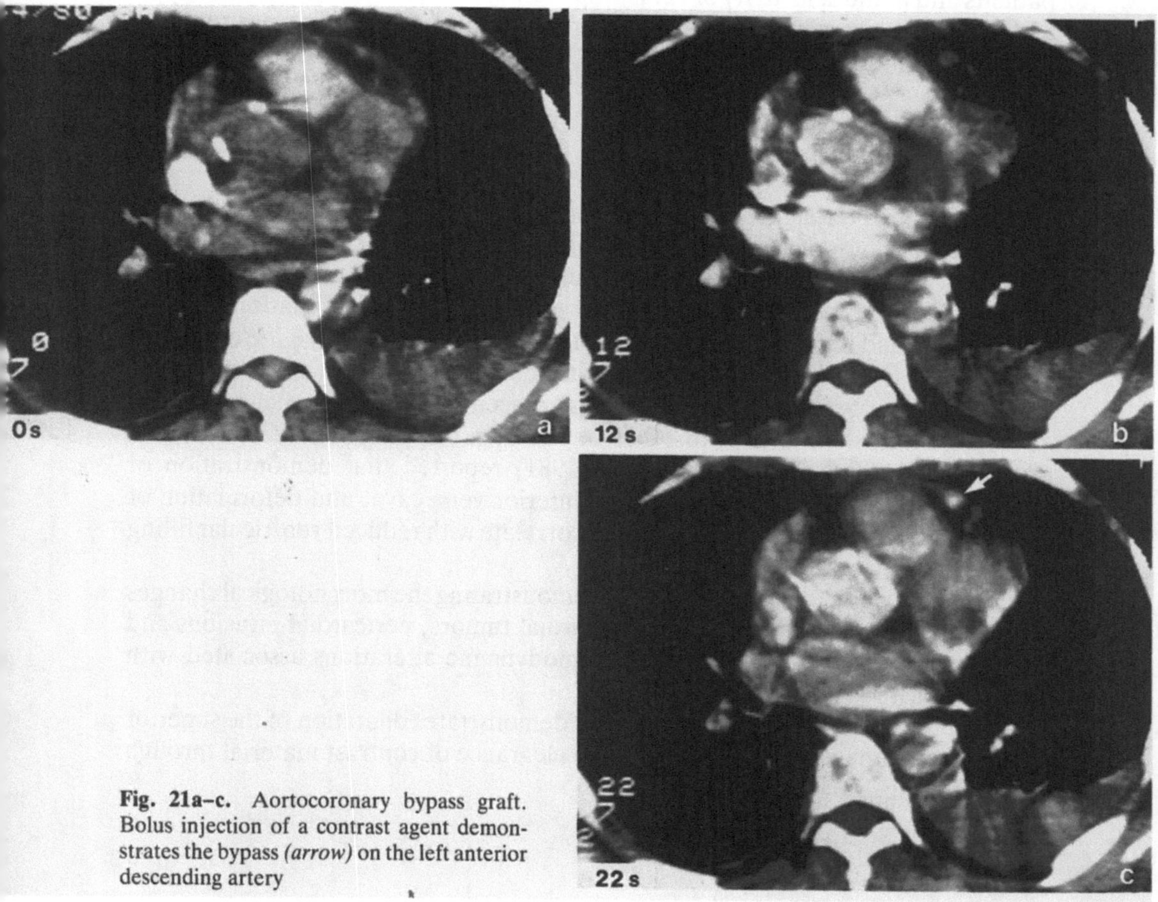

Fig. 21a–c. Aortocoronary bypass graft. Bolus injection of a contrast agent demonstrates the bypass *(arrow)* on the left anterior descending artery

graft. This method demonstrates flow of contrast medium through the graft, the right ventricle, the left ventricle and the aorta. Since the contrast medium appears in the graft slightly later than in the aorta, it is usually possible to demonstrate the graft with this method. Each CT slice requires a small amount of contrast material and this allows repeated studies in several planes.

A patent bypass graft appears as a hyperdense point after administration of a contrast medium (Fig. 21). Lackner concluded that a bypass graft may be considered patent if density increases by 30–70 HU following administration of contrast material.

Failure to demonstrate a bypass constitutes evidence that the bypass graft is not patent, but exact demonstration of the occlusion is not possible with CT studies.

Lackner et al. (1980) examined 118 patients with bypass grafts and found that CT achieved a sensitivity of 89.6% in comparison with conventional coronary angiography in the demonstration of bypass grafts, while Lipton and Higgins (1980) reported sensitivity as high as 95% in 100 patients with bypass grafts. Heuser et al. (1982) reported a multicenter study of 611 bypass grafts in 328 patients and found sensitivity of 92.6%, specificity of 78.1% and total accuracy of 87.9%. The authors concluded that interpretation of the CT findings requires knowledge of intraoperative findings.

6.2.5 Pericardial Disease

Use of CT in the diagnosis of pericardial lesions is controversial. Pericardial effusions have low density values (0–20 HU) and are easily demonstrated in plain CT scans. Loculated effusions, which cause diagnostic problems in echocardiography, are readily delineated from mediastinal lesions. Differentiation between hemorrhage and nonhemorrhagic effusions is not a problem, since the density of fresh blood is higher than that of serous fluids. CT studies are suitable for demonstration of space-occupying lesions adjacent to the pericardial cavity. CT provides a valuable adjunct to other methods in the diagnosis of constrictive pericardial disease. Doppmann et al. (1981) reported that demonstration of pericardial thickening, dilatation of the inferior vena cava, and deformation of the contours of the right or left ventricles correlate with reduced ventricular filling and stroke volume.

Dynamic CT studies are capable of demonstrating the morphological changes in constrictive pericardial disease, pericardial tumors, pericardial effusions and tamponade as well as the functional hemodynamic alterations associated with these lesions.

Administration of a contrast material demonstrates dilatation of the superior and inferior vena cava as well as delayed clearance of contrast material through the heart (Fig. 22).

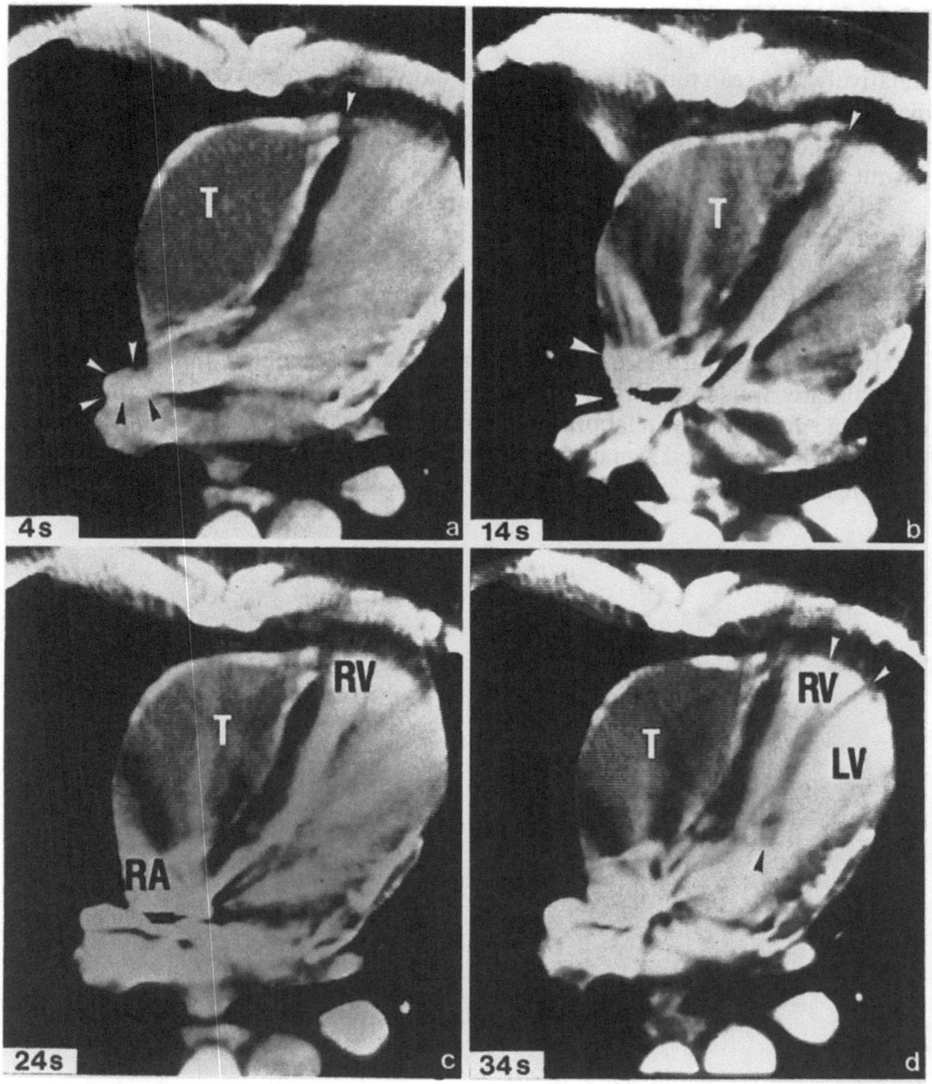

Fig. 22. **a** Pericardial space-occupying lesion with calcification *(arrow)* anterior to the right atrium and the ventricle. Density in the space-occupying lesion is 28 HU. Wide zone of pericardial calcification adjacent to the left ventricle. Delayed appearance of the contrast agent after bolus administration at the cubital vein due to pericardial constriction. Contrast enhancement of the superior vena cava *(arrows)*. **b** Initial contrast enhancement in the right ventricle *(RV)*, which is compressed by the pericardial space-occupying lesion. **c** Delayed contrast of all heart chambers. **d** Delineation of the chambers and the ventricular septum is possible only after complete contrast enhancement. Slight indentation of the left ventricle and major compression of the right ventricle. The ventricular septum *(arrow)* is deformed near the apex due to pericardial construction. The contrast agent is visible in the superior vena cava and the right atrium at 34 s. This causes contrast artifacts in the right atrium and in the superior vena cava, because the contrast agent is not diluted by blood

6.2.6 Critical Evaluation

Relatively long scan times of 3–5 s place a major limitation on the use of CT in the diagnosis of cardiac disease. Improvement in the quality of images will require a significant reduction in scan times to below 1 s, and scan times in milliseconds will permit efficient function studies of the heart.

ECG-triggered CT studies are generally performed in a single slice, and several investigators have attempted ECG-triggered studies in systole and diastole in transverse, sagittal and vertical planes in an effort at producing three-dimensional images which provide quantitative information on regional wall motion and ejection fractions.

Initial reports on the use of nuclear magnetic resonance in cardiac studies have already appeared. Brady et al. (1982) were able to demonstrate fine details of cardiac morphology in laboratory animals and to identify myocardial ischemia on the basis of reduced signal intensity in zones of infarction after administration of manganese.

6.3 Lungs and Mediastinum

CT has a distinct advantage over conventional radiologic procedures in its capacity for demonstrating anatomic relations and pathologic structures in the mediastinum in a horizontal plane without superposition of adjacent structures. However, it is often impossible to delineate a mediastinal space-occupying lesion even with the advantage of high density resolution offered by CT, which is most successful in demonstrating space-occupying lesions and vascular malformations. Use of contrast material is required in most cases.

These studies generally involve delineation of a space-occupying lesion from normal major blood vessles, which define the anatomy of the upper mediastinum. An intravenous infusion of contrast material is sufficient for this purpose in most cases. Intravascular contrast enhancement averaging 60 HU over the entire period of the examination is generally recommended. In circumscribed lesions bolus injection may occasionally prove advantageous in order to demonstrate the vascular relations of a tumor, since this may provide important information in differential diagnosis.

6.3.1 Vascular Studies

The anatomy of the mediastinum is defined by the major blood vessels. A circumscribed space-occupying lesion can be identified only when the adjacent blood vessels have been clearly demonstrated. For example, the density of a lymph node ranges from 35–50 HU and approximates that of blood. Artifacts are caused by pulsation of the vessels, with the result that current CT systems are unable to define slight differences in density. Demonstration of vascular structures also depends on the amount of fat in the mediastinum, which may be slight in thin individuals. The plane of the scan and the course of the vessel in question are also important factors in the identification of vascular structures. Axial projections are usually more valuable than tangential slices for identification of a vessel. Contrast enhancement of approximately 60 HU permits unequivocal demonstration of the aortic arch, the ascending and descending aorta, the origins of the major vessels and the superior vena cava. It is also possible to visualize the innominate vein, the internal jugular vein, the origin of the subclavian vein, the common carotid artery, the pulmonary artery and the azygos vein.

6.3.2 Vascular Anomalies and Tumors in the Mediastinum

Dynamic CT demonstrates congenital anomalies of the major mediastinal vessels with a high degree of accuracy and without resort to conventional angiography. Baron at al. (1981) reported successful visualization of the superior vena cava, a right aortic arch with aberrant left subclavian artery, transposition of the great vessels, stenoses, and truncus arteriosus in the absence of the right pulmonary artery. Diagnosis with dynamic CT is sometimes made as a result of altered temporal relationships in enhancement of the major vessels.

Delineation of a space-occupying lesion raises the question of the nature of the lesion. Location of the lesion within the mediastinum provides important information, and analysis of density values in the plain scan adds to the diagnostic yield.

Bolus injection of contrast material shows the vascularity of the space-occupying lesion. If the tumor contains no blood vessels, the amount of protein within the lesion is of interest. Hematomas, abscesses and bronchogenic cysts have density values of approximately 30 HU and cannot be differentiated from solid lesions without resort to contrast media. Failure to enhance suggests the presence of a cystic lesion. There have been few reports in the literature to date on characteristic vascularization patterns in specific tumors (Fig. 23). A mediastinal space-occupying lesion which proved to be a papillary thyroid carcinoma showed delayed contrast enhancement which attained a maximum of 50 HU at 50 s after contrast administration. Density within the tumor declined at the same rate as that in the aorta (Fig. 24).

A malignant thymoma in our series showed slight enhancement, approximately 20 HU (Fig. 25).

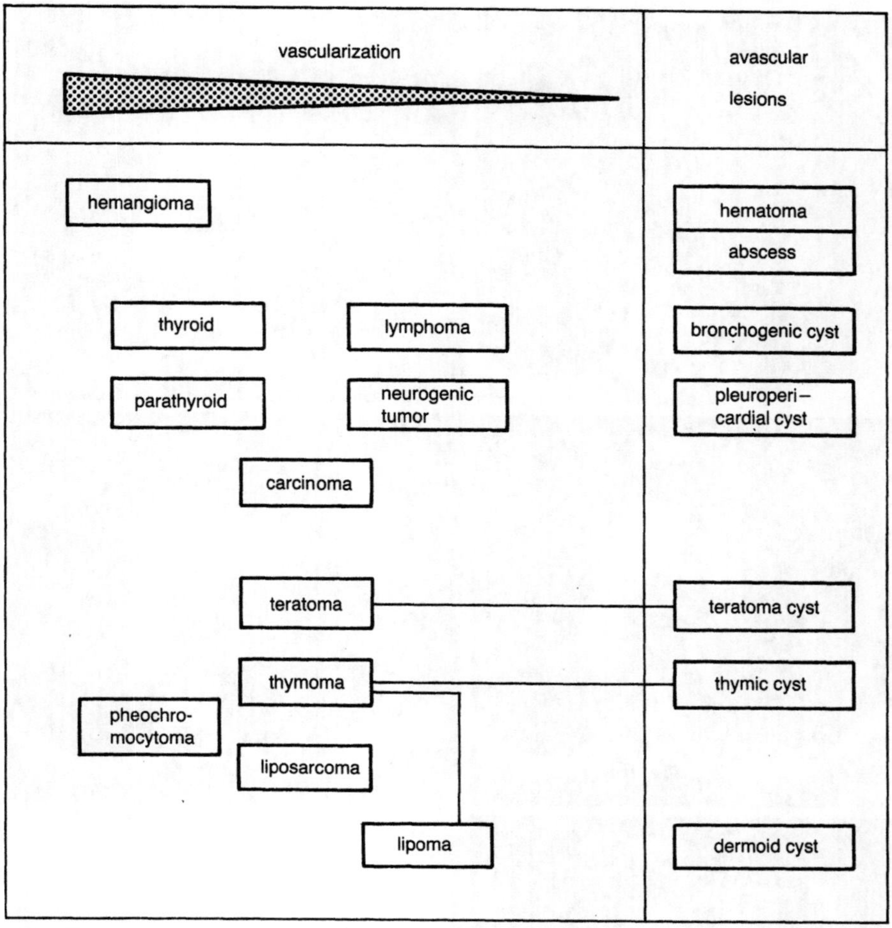

Fig. 23. Origin and degree of vascularization of mediastinal tumors (after Wegener and Claussen 1981)

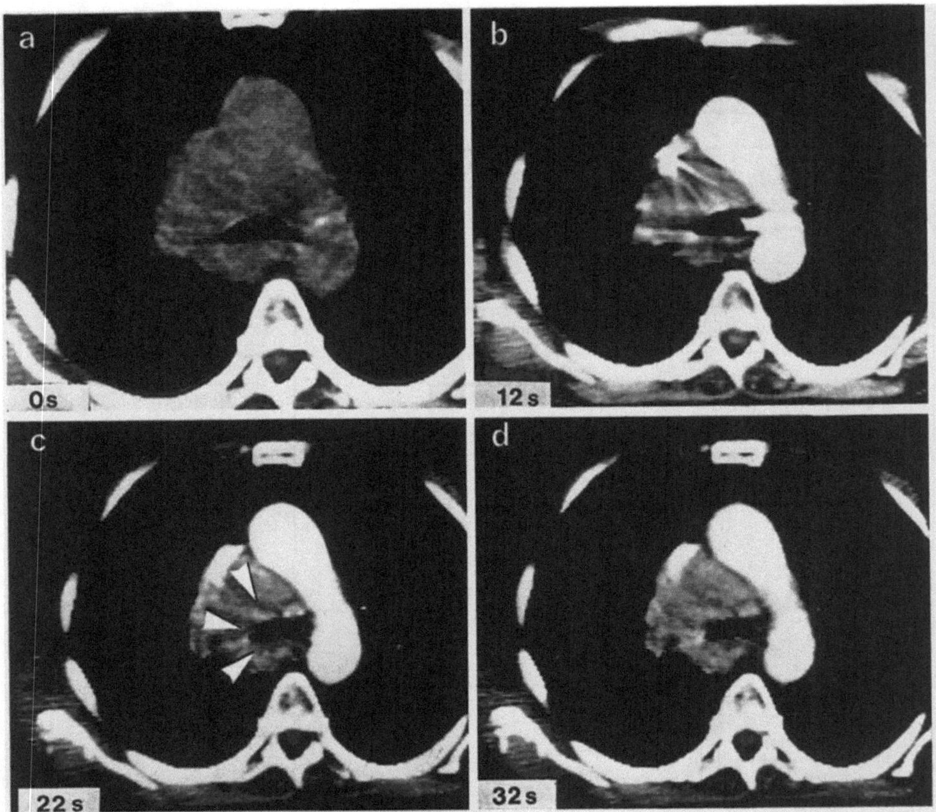

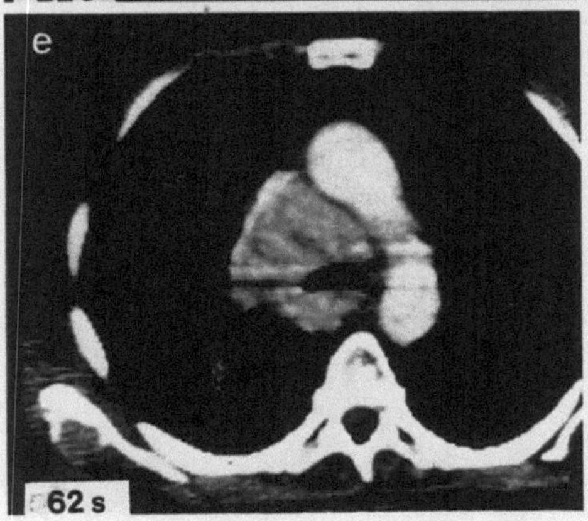

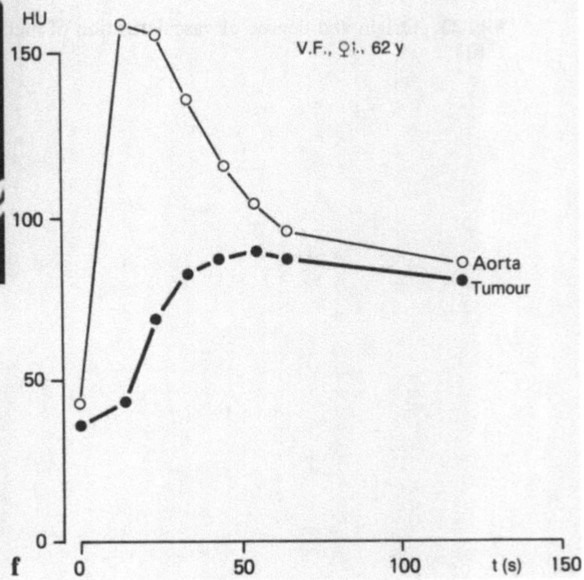

Fig. 24a–f. Papillary thyroid carcinoma with extension to the anterior mediastinum. A poorly defined isodense space-occupying lesion is demonstrated slightly to the right of and anterior to the trachea in the plain CT scan. Contrast enhancement shows the tumor which extends past the trachea on the right and enhances rather late *(arrows)*

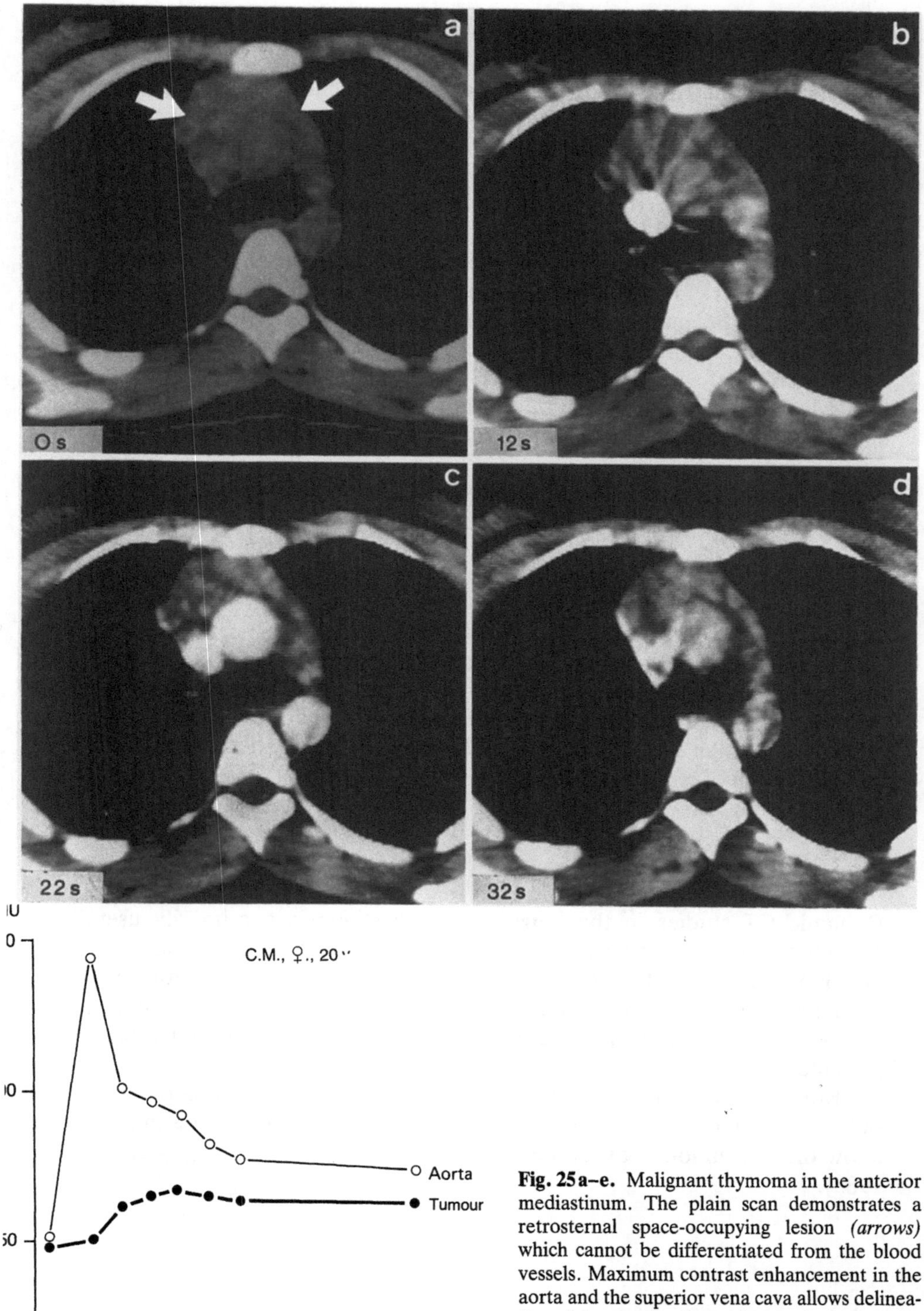

Fig. 25 a–e. Malignant thymoma in the anterior mediastinum. The plain scan demonstrates a retrosternal space-occupying lesion *(arrows)* which cannot be differentiated from the blood vessels. Maximum contrast enhancement in the aorta and the superior vena cava allows delineation of the poorly enhanced tumor in the anterior mediastinum

6.3.3 Pulmonary and Pleural Tumors

Reports on use of dynamic CT in the diagnosis of pulmonary and pleural space-occupying lesions have been rather rare. Godwin and Webb (1981) concluded that the chief value of dynamic CT lies in differentiation between vascular and nonvascular tumors. The authors report that time-density curves are useful in differentiating between tumors supplied by the pulmonary artery and those in the systemic arterial bed.

This information is significant in planning surgical strategy. A coin lesion with extreme contrast enhancement raises suspicion of an arteriovenous fistula with distension of the pulmonary veins. Inflammation generally results in slight contrast enhancement. Neoplasms, especially bronchial carcinomas, show moderate contrast enhancement, and central zones of necrosis may be demonstrated. Centrally located tumors near the aorta can be identified when the lesion is delineated against the aorta, which simultaneously excludes the diagnosis of aortic aneurysm (Fig. 26).

It is also possible to differentiate between other solid space-occupying lesions such as lymphomas in the hilum and large vessels.

Small coin lesions within the lung itself are a problem, since the partial volume effect and respiratory motion result in such inaccuracy that it is impossible to obtain valid time-density curves.

Pleural mesotheliomas have maximum contrast enhancement averaging 70 HU; approximately the same values are found in extensive pleural scarring, so that differentiation between these lesions is not possible with dynamic CT. Contrast enhancement is useful in differentiating a solid lesion from a pleural effusion with high protein content, and certain differentiation usually requires administration of contrast material.

6.3.4 Critical Evaluation

Dynamic CT studies in the lungs and mediastinum are primarily useful in discriminating between vascular and nonvascular space-occupying lesions. It is possible to differentiate between a vascular anomaly, an aortic aneurysm and a solid mediastinal tumor without resort to conventional angiography. Delineation of vascular structures from solid or cystic avascular lesions in the hilum is also possible.

Bolus injection of a contrast agent enables one to discriminate between a pulmonary tumor and surrounding collapsed lung parenchyma. This in turn may allow differentiation between benign and malignant atelectasis (Naidich et al. 1983).

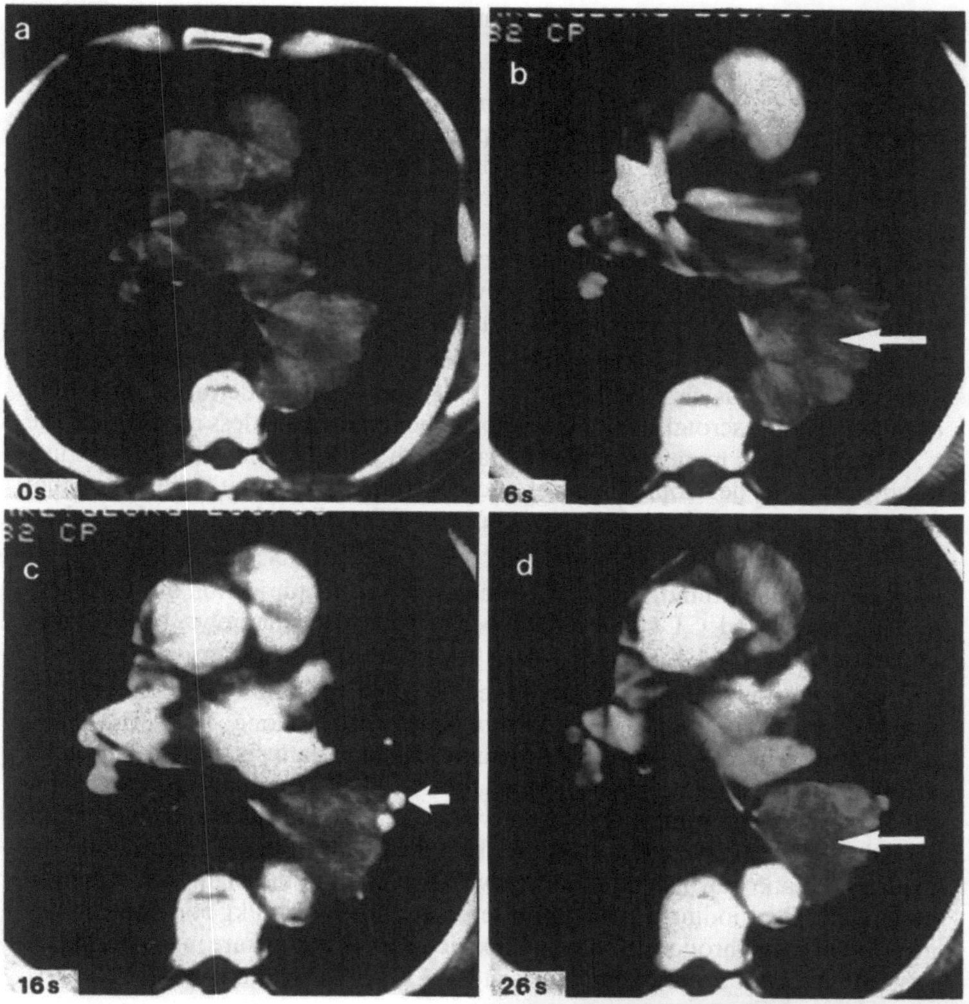

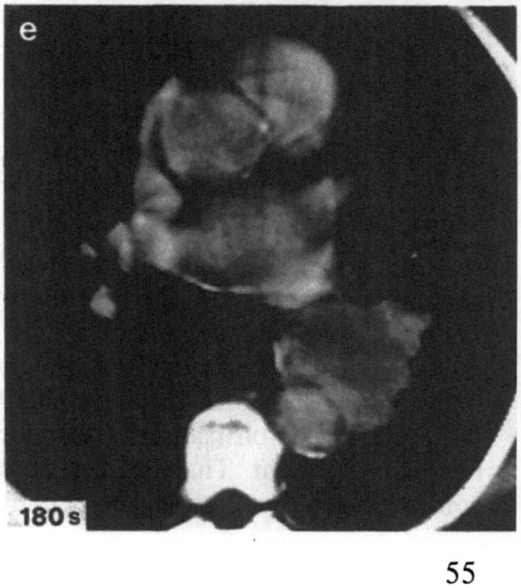

Fig. 26a–e. Central bronchial carcinoma (G.A., male, 81 years). The precontrast scan shows a space-occupying lesion measuring 5×4 cm which is located superior and dorsal to the left hilum of the lung; the lesion is not clearly delineated against the descending aorta. An aneurysm was also considered as a possible diagnosis. Administration of a contrast agent allows clear delineation of the tumor, which demonstrates low contrast enhancement. Displacement of the pulmonary arteries *(arrows)* in the periphery of the lesion is visible at 16 s after bolus injection

6.4 Experimental Hepatic Neoplasms

Experiments were performed in laboratory animals to determine whether isodense tumors which do not appear in plain CT scans can be visualized with the help of bolus injection of a contrast medium. Burgener and Violante (1979) and Violante and Dean (1980) were the first to report on demonstration of VX2 tumors introduced into the rabbit liver by intravenous (portal vein), intra-arterial, or direct intraparenchymal injection. Intravascular introduction of tumor cells is followed by diffuse growth throughout the liver, while direct implantation results in a circumscribed tumor.

We chose the Brown-Pearce tumor for our experimental studies in rabbits. This neoplasm was first described in 1923 and is an epidermoid carcinoma originating in the scrotal skin of the rabbit. The tumor grows less rapidly than the VX2 lesion, and metastases appear later. The VX2 tumor has the distinct disadvantage of developing central necrosis rather early, with the result that metastases appear as hypodense structures in CT studies after a relatively short period of growth.

Circumscribed tumor growth was achieved by direct injection of tumor cells into the liver, and CT studies were performed approximately 3 weeks after implantation.

Since central necrosis is very limited, it is not possible to demonstrate the tumor in the plain CT scan on the basis of density values alone. The entire liver is demonstrated in plain scans before dynamic CT studies are performed. The latter are made in a plane at the point at which tumor cells were initially introduced into the liver, since the tumor itself is not visible in the plain scan and since tumor growth is most likely at this location. This means that dynamic CT studies are made in a plane in which no tumor growth is evident in the plain scan. Contrast material (300 mg iodine/ml) is administered in a dose of 2 ml/kg body weight over a period of 1–2 s through an ear vein. Six pictures per minute are made during the first minute, with subsequent studies at 90, 120, 240, 300, and 600 s.

Dynamic CT studies demonstrate maximum contrast enhancement in normal liver tissue between 15 and 40 s after contrast administration, while there is no evident enhancement in the tumor, which is sharply delineated against normal adjacent liver tissue. Further studies up to 600 s following administration of the contrast medium demonstrate a decline in contrast enhancement within normal tissue, which results in a reduced gradient between normal tissue and the neoplasm (Fig. 27).

Low contrast enhancement in the tumor is most evident at the time of maximum contrast flow and is primarily related to blood flow within the tumor. There is little contrast uptake in the tumor in later phases, which results in reduced contrast between the tumor and adjacent normal tissue as density values in the latter fall. Violante and Dean (1980) demonstrated that contrast media are required for demonstration of a tumor less than 1 cm in diameter if little or no necrosis is present. Their studies were performed with intravenous infusion of contrast media but without the benefit of time-density analysis.

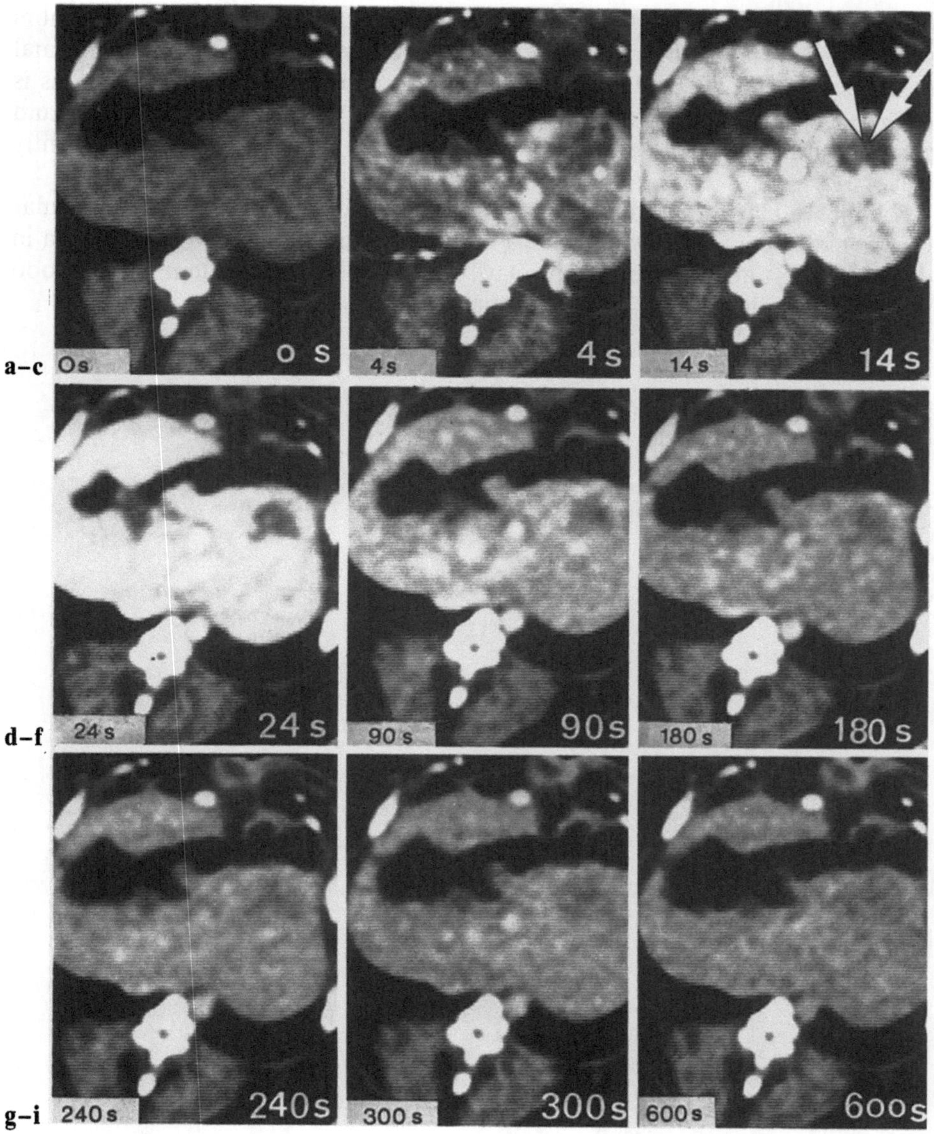

Fig. 27a–i. Demonstration of a Brown-Pearce tumor implanted in the liver of a rabbit. Serial CT scans of the liver with contrast enhancement demonstrate a tumor 1×2 cm in diameter not visible in the plain scan but clearly defined at the moment of maximum contrast enhancement. (Claussen et al. 1983b)

The results achieved with dynamic CT studies in experimental liver tumors show that maximum contrast between isodense tumors and surrounding normal tissue is attained within the first minute after contrast administration. This is followed by gradual equalization of density values within the tumor and surrounding tissue, and isodense tumors without necrotic zones subsequently disappear.

Improved contrast and demonstration of hypovascular and avascular intrahepatic space-occupying lesions after bolus injection of contrast media in dynamic CT studies are related primarily to contrast enhancement within blood vessels rather than in the interstitial space.

6.5 Liver

Density values in the human liver average 60 HU (61.3 ± 11.6 HU as reported by Hübener).

Demonstration of a hepatic space-occupying lesion depends on the presence of a contrast gradient between the lesion and surrounding normal tissue. Most hepatic lesions are visible in plain CT scans as a result of low density values, but reduced density within liver tissue secondary to fatty infiltration or other forms of diffuse liver disease may result in decreased contrast between a tumor and nonneoplastic tissue within the liver. Hepatic metastases may be overlooked in cases of diffuse fatty infiltration of the liver. When density values within the liver are 15 HU lower than normal or serum liver enzymes are elevated, dynamic CT studies should be performed in several planes for clarification of questionable pathologic findings obtained with diagnostic ultrasound or scintigraphy.

Density values may be lower at the centre than at the periphery of a hepatic metastasis or primary liver cell carcinoma, and serial CT studies aid in providing a clearer line of demarcation between the intrahepatic space-occupying lesion and normal tissue. Intravenous administration of a contrast agent has the additional advantage of demonstrating the vascularity of the tumor itself, though CT studies are inferior to conventional angiography in most cases in demonstrating the vascular relations of the tumor.

Time-density analysis reveals the vascularity of an intrahepatic space-occupying lesion in the early phase of the study up to 60 s and in later stages as well. Avascular tumors are best demonstrated by virtue of an increased contrast gradient resulting from contrast enhancement in normal tissue, which attains a maximum during transit of the contrast medium in the portal circulation. Strong enhancement immediately after administration followed by a rapid drop in density values within a circumscribed lesion suggests the presence of a highly vascular tumor, as is also the case in conventional angiographic studies.

6.5.1 Vascular Studies

The portal and hepatic veins appear as round and elongated hypodense structures in the plain CT scan. Examination of several adjacent slices usually allows ready identification of the portal veins by virtue of their relations to the hilum and of the hepatic veins on the basis of their relations to the vena cava (Fig. 28). The vessels are not visible in cases of fatty infiltration of the liver with a reduction in density of 20–30 HU in the plain scan. The bile ducts are found parallel to the portal vessels but are usually not visible unless biliary contrast media are used, except in cases of significant dilatation of the ducts. The major branches of the hepatic artery are easily identified as a result of high contrast enhancement in the early phase and readily differentiated from portal veins, which appear hypodense at this time (Fig. 28). The portal veins enhance at 20–40 s after contrast administration (Figs. 28, 29a). Round or slightly elongated hypodense structures near the vena cava which demonstrate slight enhancement still later are the hepatic veins (Fig. 28).

The temporal relations of contrast enhancement in the hepatic arteries, portal veins and hepatic veins were defined in 92 dynamic CT studies (Fig. 29b).

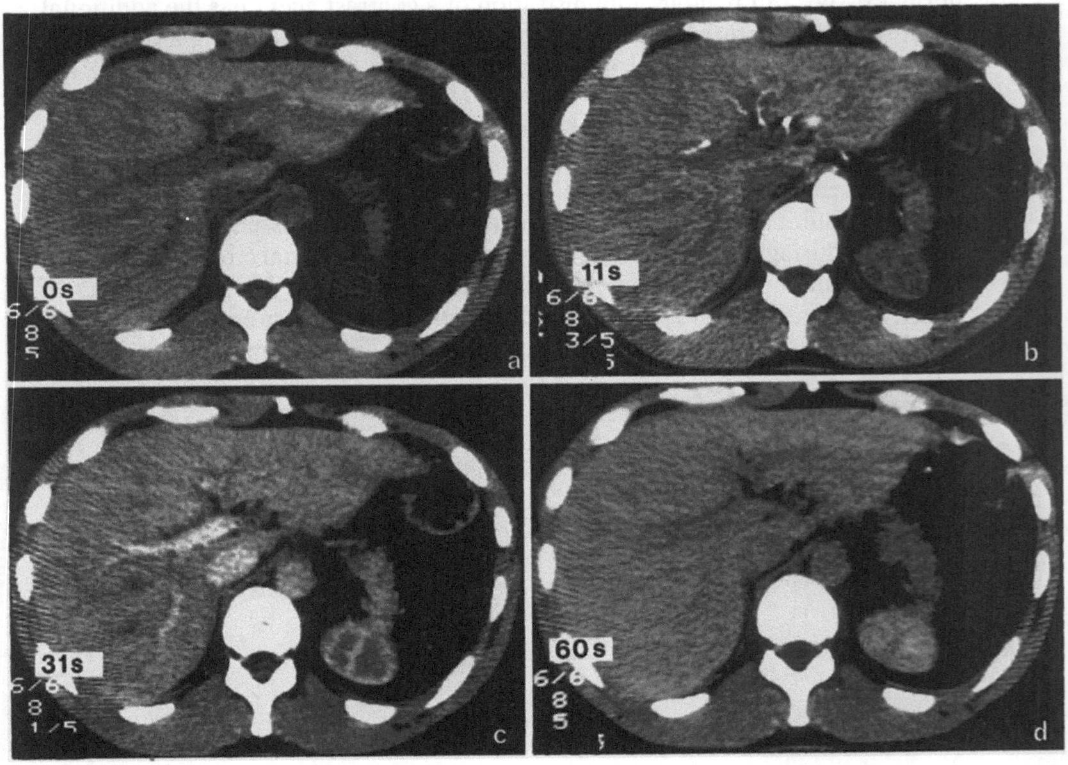

Fig. 28a–d. Dynamic CT studies of the liver with demonstration of the hepatic vessels after intravenous administration of the contrast agent. **a** Plain CT study. **b** Contrast enhancement in the aorta and the arteries near the hilum of the liver at 11 s. **c** Significant enhancement in the portal veins at 31 s; the hypodense structures are hepatic veins. **d** Homogeneous contrast enhancement within the entire liver at 60 s

Fig. 29. **a** Time-density diagram of the hepatic vessels after intravenous administration of a contrast agent, based on the average values. **b** Contrast enhancement of the hepatic vessels after bolus injection of a contrast agent ($n = 92$)

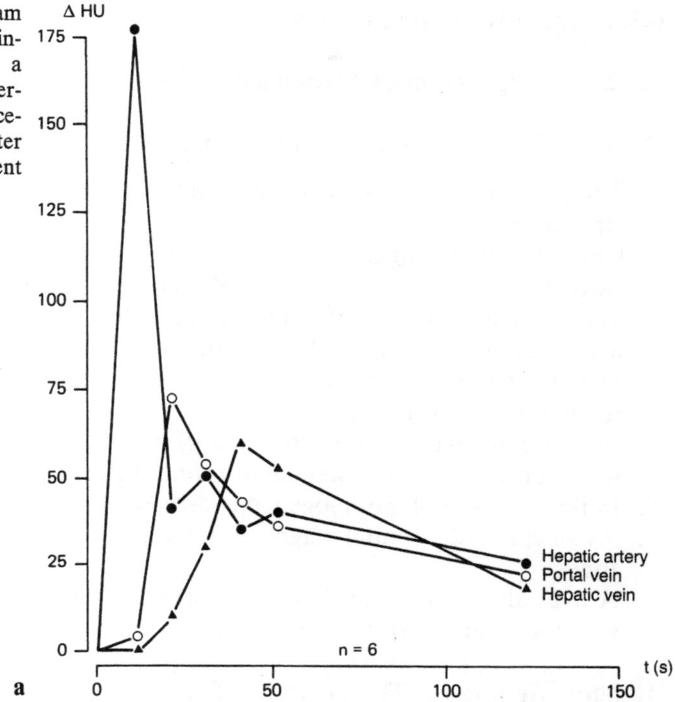

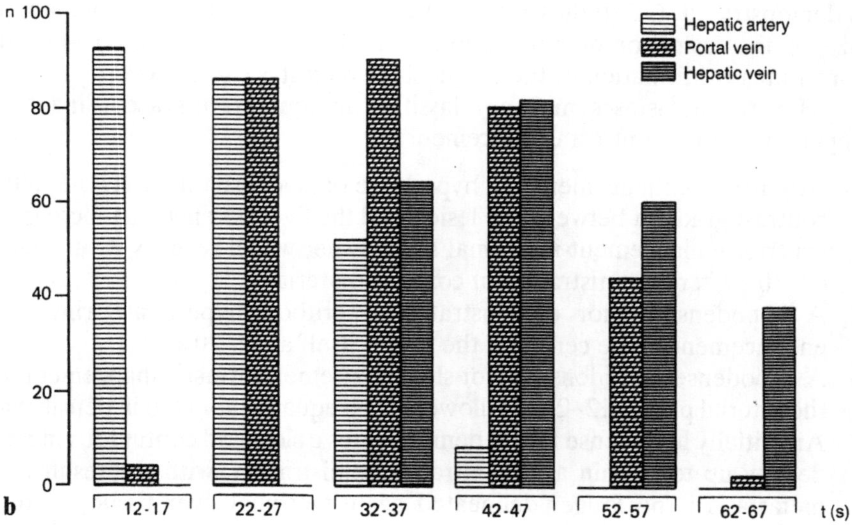

6.5.2 Space-Occupying Lesions

6.5.2.1 Malignant Space-Occupying Lesions

Dynamic CT studies of the liver are performed in the following circumstances:

1. The plain scan reveals one or more hypodense zones not related to vascular structures.
2. Clinical findings suggest the presence of liver metastases or a primary liver carcinoma, for example, in cases of gross changes in the size or shape of the liver, or in the presence of increased values for α_1-fetoprotein even when there are no circumscribed or diffuse changes in density in the plain scan.
3. Hepatic metastases are suspected and the plain scan demonstrates a diffuse reduction in density values.
4. In order to exclude the presence of additional lesions prior to planned resection when a single hypodense zone suggests a solitary metastasis.
5. In the presence of inhomogeneous density values in one or more lobes.
6. As an aid in differential diagnosis in the presence of one or more hypodense zones.
7. A liver abscess is suspected and a circumscribed hypodense zone or region with the same density as water is found.

Hepatic Metastases. The presence of hypodense zones in the plain scan in a patient with a known primary tumor and pathologic serum enzymes suggests a diagnosis of metastasis in the liver. When a single lesion less than 2 cm in diameter is demonstrated, CT studies are repeated at 3 and 6 months. An increase in the size of the lesion or demonstration of multiple lesions in follow-up studies constitutes confirmation of the diagnosis of metastasis to the liver.

Hepatic metastases may be classified in four groups according to their appearance after contrast enhancement:

1. Absence of enhancement in a hypodense or isodense tumor (HU 5–30). The contrast gradient between the lesion and the liver parenchyma increases with contrast enhancement in normal liver tissue, which reaches its maximum at 40–50 s after administration of contrast material.
2. A hypodense tumor demonstrates a perifocal hyperdense ring without enhancement in the centre of the tumor itself at 12–70 s.
3. A hypodense or isodense tumor shows extreme contrast enhancement during the arterial phase (12–22 s) followed by an equally rapid fall in density values.
4. An initially hypodense tumor demonstrates a slow and continuous increase in density up to 10 min after contrast administration, with the result that the metastasis is no longer delineated against normal liver tissue, a so-called vanishing lesion. This type of contrast enhancement is caused by diffusion of contrast medium into the interstitial space of the tumor itself.

Ring enhancement in group 2 is related to hypervascularization in the periphery of a metastasis and may appear at various times after contrast administration. Some lesions demonstrate maximum enhancement in the arterial

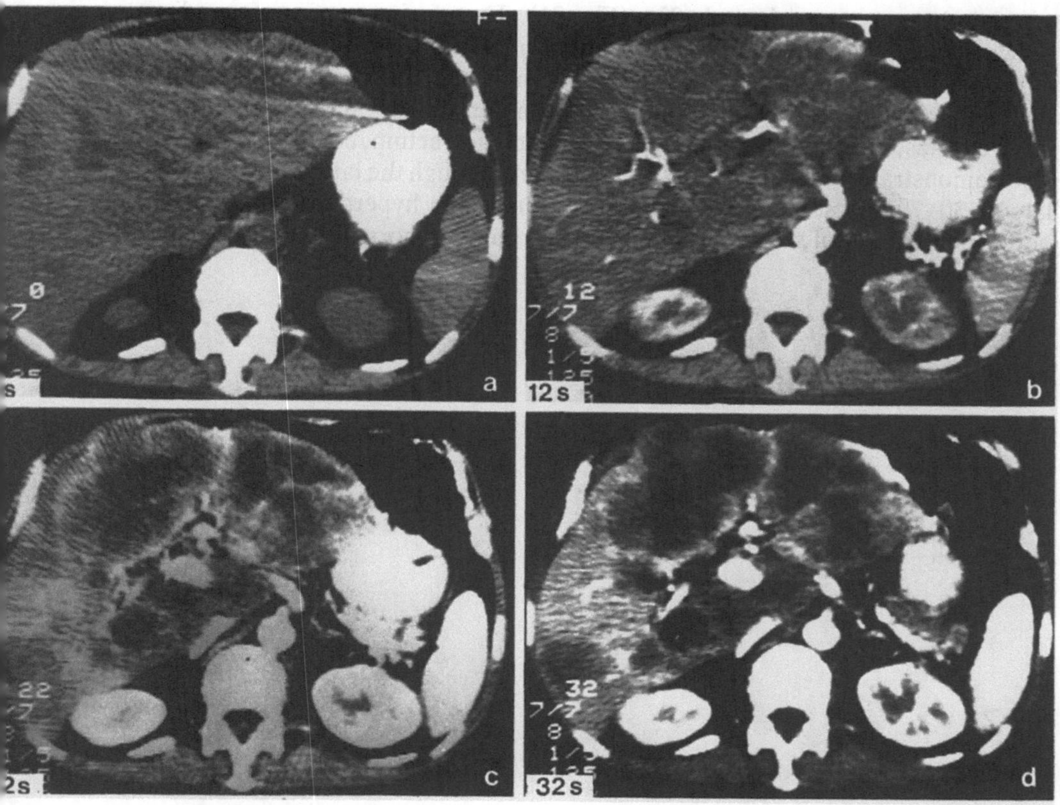

Fig. 30a–d. Metastases of prostatic carcinoma (A.J., male, 74 years). The plain CT scan demonstrates irregular enlargement of the liver without circumscribed lesions, suggesting metastases. The small oval and elongated hypodense areas are vascular structures. Contrast enhancement **(b–d)** delineates the large metastases

phase at 12–32 s, while others have a maximum in the portal phase at 22–32 s and are still evident at 70 s after contrast administration.

The findings described in group 1 are demonstrated in almost all metastases of bronchial carcinoma, and in the majority of hepatic lesions in prostate and breast cancer (Fig. 30). Many gastrointestinal tumors have metastases with the characteristics described in group 2. All metastases produced by carcinoma of the esophagus demonstrate a hyperdense ring lesion which is most pronounced in the arterial phase at approximately 22 s (Fig. 31). The maximum contrast gradient between the malignant lesion and adjacent normal liver tissue is 20–25 HU at 22 s after injection. The contrast ring is scarcely visible at 120 s. The central region of the metastasis only rarely shows an increase in density of 5–8 HU.

Metastases of adenocarcinomas of the pancreas, rectum, colon, and stomach also demonstrate a ring of contrast enhancement, though the latter may appear as late as 30–70 s in some cases. Demonstration of the hyperdense ring permits better delineation of the metastasis from surrounding normal liver tissue in all cases.

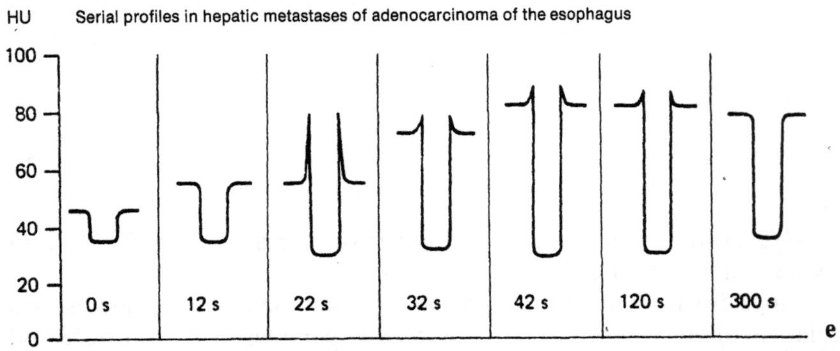

Fig. 31a–e. Hepatic metastases of carcinoma of the esophagus (W. F., 58 years). **a** Several indistinctly defined hypodense zones are visible at the periphery of the right hepatic lobe in the plain CT scan. **b** There is a peripheral ring of contrast enhancement surrounding the hypodense structures at 32 s

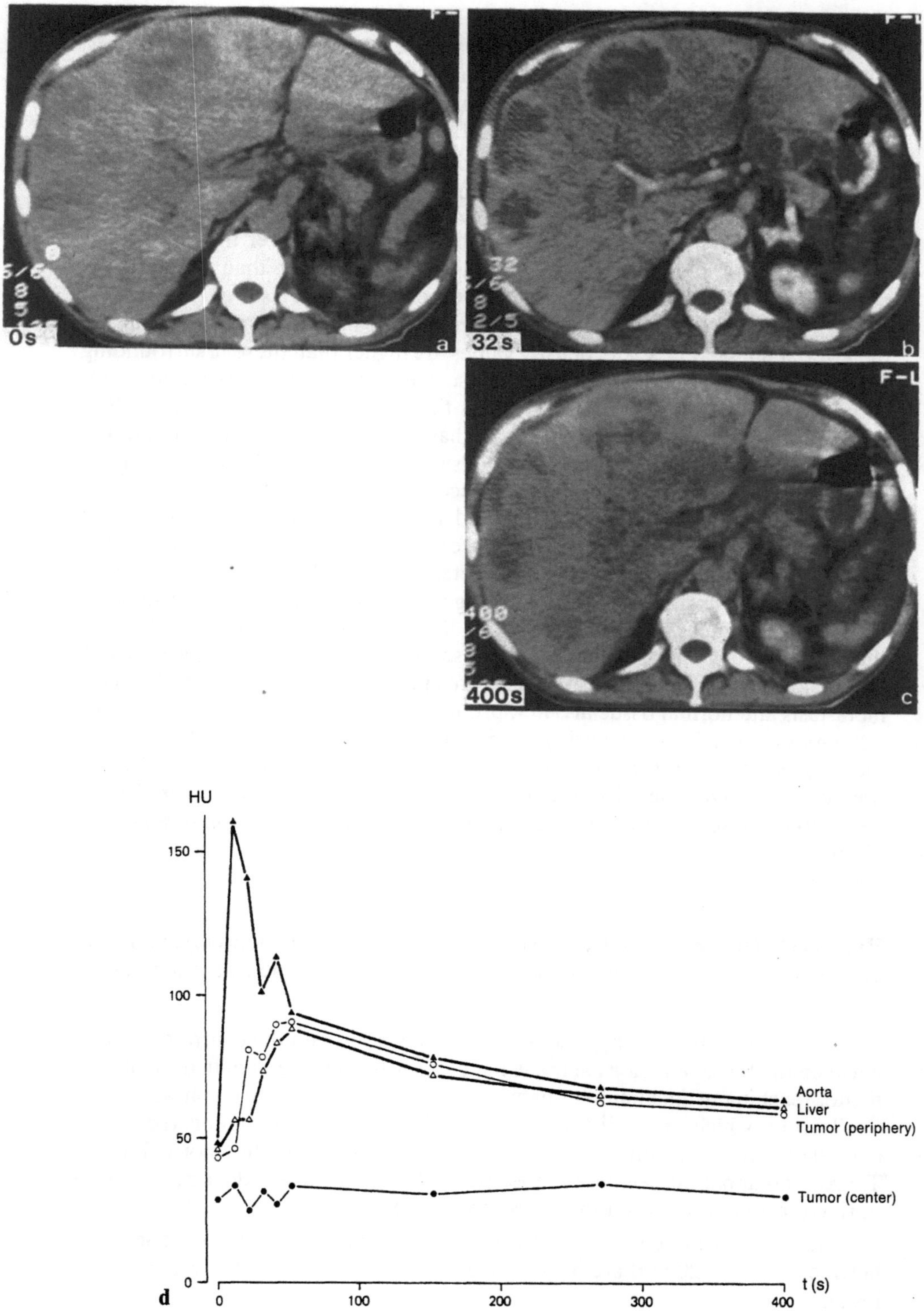
0s
a
32s
b
400s
c
HU
150
100
50
0
Aorta
Liver
Tumor (periphery)
Tumor (center)
t (s)
0
100
200
300
400
d

The type of contrast enhancement described in group 3 is often found in metastases of renal carcinoma. There is extreme contrast enhancement during the arterial phase due to considerable vascularity in the metastasis, while zones of necrosis in large metastases fail to enhance. Metastases of renal carcinomas sometimes demonstrate isodense values in the plain scan (Fig. 32). There is strong enhancement in the arterial phase at 12–22 s after administration of contrast material, followed by a decrease in density in the hyperdense zone at 32 s. The lesion is generally isodense once again at 120 s, and the further decline in density values within the metastasis parallels that in surrounding liver tissue. In some cases the metastases have density values 15–25 HU lower than the adjacent normal liver tissue, as is the case in many other hepatic metastases (Fig. 32).

In this type of metastasis in hypernephroma the same flush is observed during the arterial phase at 22 s, and density values are higher than those in surrounding liver tissue at 50 s. The subsequent decrease in enhancement is rapid, and values within the metastasis average 20 HU less than in adjacent tissue at 120–180 s (Fig. 32). The rapid decrease in contrast enhancement after the arterial phase and the decline to hypodense values thereafter suggest that there is limited passage of contrast medium into the interstitial space of the tumor. Metastases of carcinomas originating in the lung, colon and stomach are initially hypodense and demonstrate a slow and continuous increase in contrast enhancement over 10 min (group 4). Density values within the metastases, which are often indistinctly delineated from normal liver tissue, average 20 HU lower than those in adjacent liver parenchyma, and the increase within the lesion is only about 15 HU during the first minute. Contrast enhancement is somewhat delayed in comparison with that in normal tissue, and density values are approximately equal at 65 HU in the metastasis and normal tissue at 300 s, producing so-called vanishing lesions. The latter may escape detection during continuous infusion of contrast material due to the passage of contrast medium into the interstitial space of the tumor. Precontrast scans and dynamic CT studies with bolus injection of contrast material aid in delineating these lesions during the phase of strong contrast enhancement at 40–50 s.

Hepatocellular carcinoma. Contrast enhancement following bolus injection may be classified into four groups similar to those presented in the discussion of liver metastases.

Type 1. The tumor is hypodense in the plain scan, and the contrast gradient between the tumor and normal tissue increases with enhancement in normal liver tissue, reaching its maximum at between 40 and 50 s in the portal phase.

Tumors which are indistinct in the plain scan are well delineated in the contrast study as a result of the increased density in surrounding normal tissue. There is no apparent decrease in the size of the tumor, which does not enhance during the 10 min required for the contrast study (Table 2).

Type 2. A hypodense tumor demonstrates a ring of contrast enhancement between 32 and 120 s; there is no change in density values at the centre of the lesion.

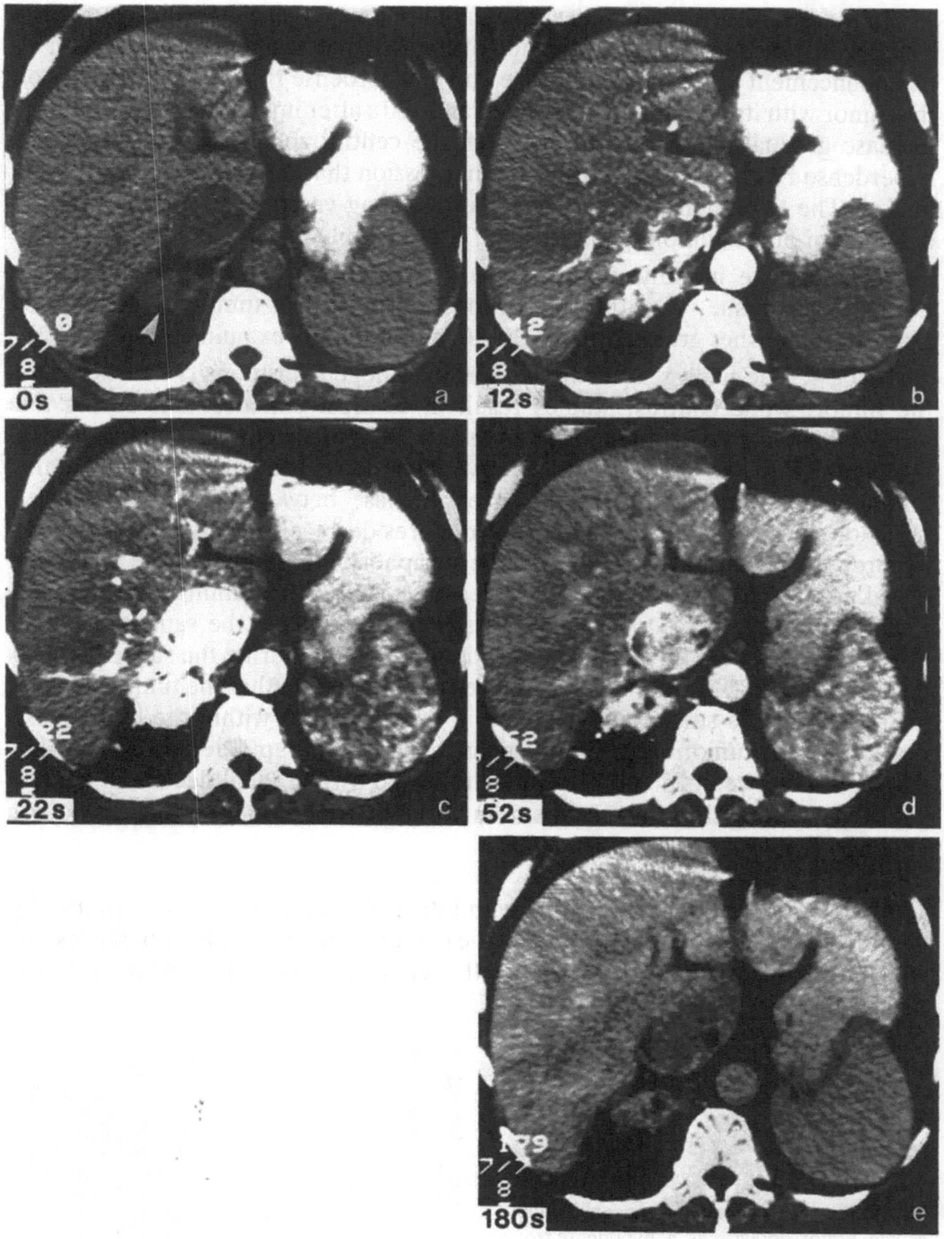

Fig. 32a–e. Metastasis of renal carcinoma (J. S., 61 years) in the caudate lobe with entrapment and infiltration of the vena cava and metastasis in the right adrenal gland *(arrow)*. Significant contrast enhancement at **b** 12 s and **c** 22 s. **e** Findings similar to those in the precontrast study at 180 s

In these cases the plain scan shows an inhomogeneous, generally hypodense lesion with indistinct borders. Injection of contrast material results in characteristic enhancement in normal liver tissue and a hyperdense ring at the periphery of the tumor with its maximum between 30 and 120 s after injection. Density values increase gradually in the tissue between the central zone of necrosis and the hyperdense ring, and this produces the impression that the tumor has decreased in size. The hyperdense zone is not due to strong vascularity but allows good delineation of the tumor against normal tissue (Table 2).

Type 3. The initially isodense lesion accepts less contrast material than normal liver tissue, resulting in demonstration of the tumor. The contrast gradient diminishes gradually over the 10 min of the CT examination (Table 2).

Type 4. The plain scan demonstrates inhomogeneous density values within the tumor, while contrast studies result in contrast enhancement during the arterial phase in initially hypodense areas as a result of irregular vascularization in the tumor (Fig. 33a–d). Multiple hypervascular zones become visible within the inhomogeneous tumor during the arterial phase between 12 and 22 s after injection, and density values in these structures decrease rapidly after 40 s. The hyperdense areas may be found in the periphery of the hypodense tumor or distributed irregularly throughout the lesion, sometimes attaining a diameter of 2 cm (Fig. 33b). At 45 s the highly vascular lesions have the same density as normal liver tissue, and no contrast gradient is evident during the subsequent 10 min of the study (Fig. 33d). This produces the impression that the tumor declines in size during the study. The decrease in density values within the hyperdense portions of the tumor occurs in two phases. The initial rapid decrease in density takes place between 25 and 40 s and is followed by a gradual decline in density values paralleling the decrease found in normal tissue. Zones of necrosis do not enhance (Table 2).

Cholangioma. Bile duct carcinoma with intrahepatic extension does not usually demonstrate contrast enhancement at the center or in the periphery of the lesion, which is slightly hypodense and indistictly delineated against normal tissue in the plain scan (Fig. 34).

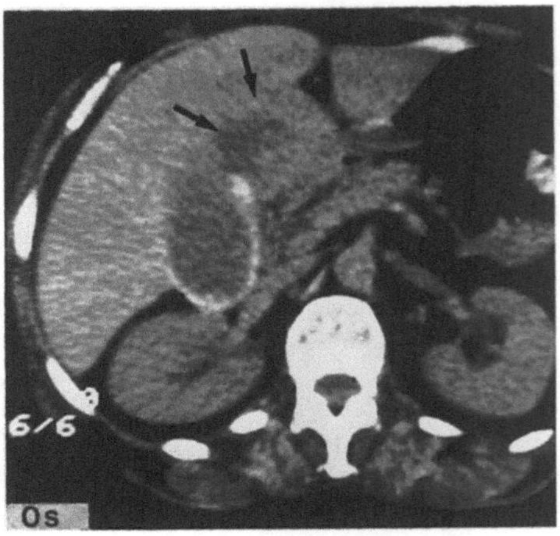

a

Fig. 34a–c. Carcinoma of the gallbladder. **a** The tumor appears as a hypodense zone invading the quadrate lobe *(arrows)* in the plain scan. **b** Extensive infiltration of the quadrate lobe is fully demonstrated in the early phase of contrast enhancement. Infiltrative growth of the tumor results in inhomogeneous perfusion within the liver *(arrows)*. **c** As in the plain scan, the tumor appears hypodense in late studies but is more clearly delineated against normal liver tissue

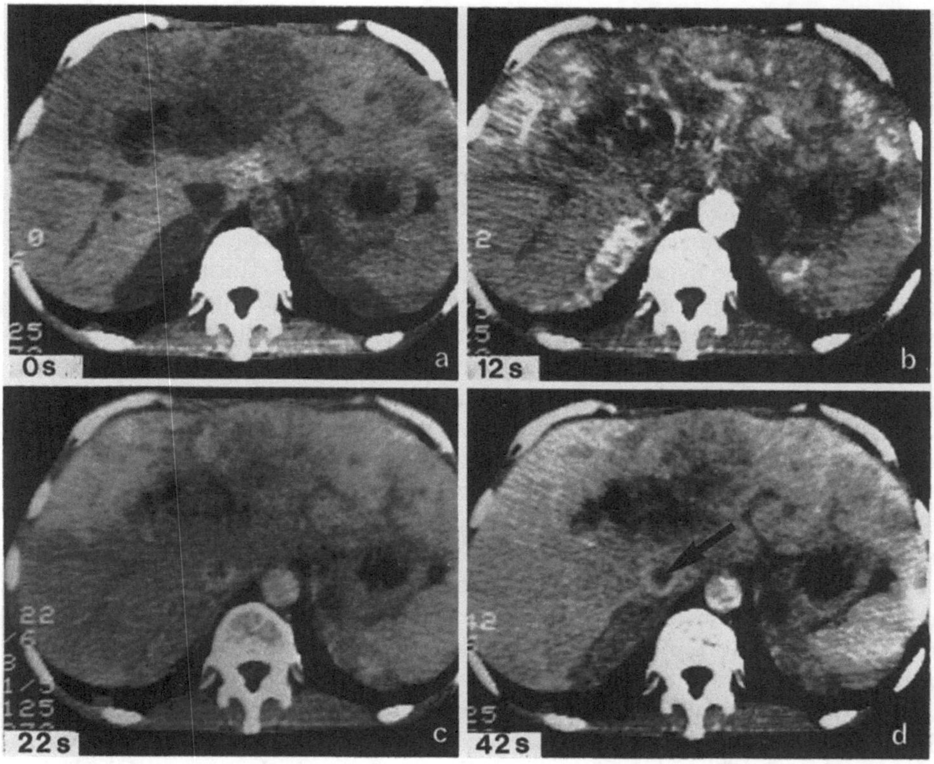

Fig. 33a–d. Hepatocellular carcinoma (type 4) (C. S., 52 years). Hypervascular structures are irregularly distributed throughout the right and left hepatic lobes at 12 s. There is a rapid decrease in density values thereafter (cf. time-density curves in Table 3). Thrombosis of the vena cava *(arrow)*

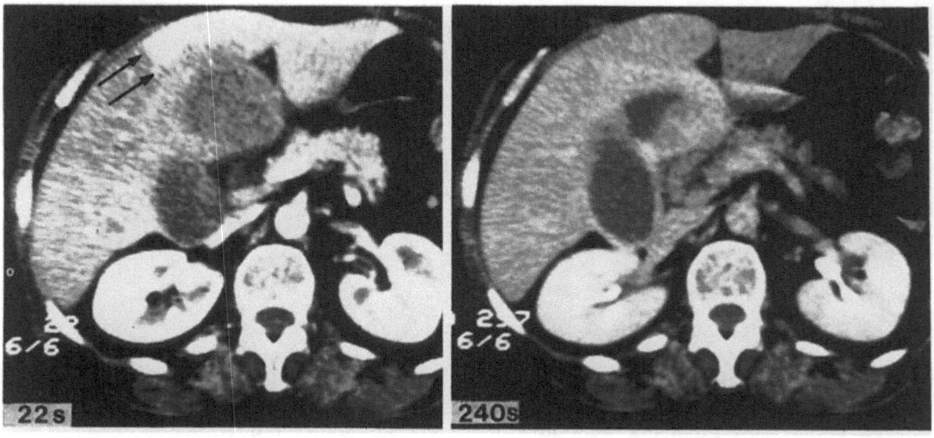

b **c**

6.5.2.2 Benign Hepatic Lesions

Cavernous hemangioma. Cavernous hemangiomas in the liver usually appear as sharply delineated hyperdense zones with density values approximately 20–25 HU lower than adjacent hepatic tissue in the plain CT scan.

There is significant contrast enhancement in the periphery of the hyperdense lesion at 12 s (Fig. 35). Hypervascularization is irregular, and contrast enhancement is most pronounced near the hilum of the liver in most cases. There is no enhancement in the hypodense center of the lesion in the arterial phase. At 22 s there is a continuous increase in density values which results in an apparent reduction in the size of the hypodense lesion, while the initially hypodense center of the tumor demonstrates a gradual increase in density values. At 2 min the center of the lesion demonstrates the same density values as normal liver tissue, while the hyperdense ring visible in the first minute is no longer evident. Density values in the liver, the hemangioma, and the aorta are identical at 180 s (Fig. 35). Slightly hypodense values appear in a lesion between 5 and 10 min following contrast administration, with values approximately 12–14 HU lower than in adjacent liver tissue at 10 min.

As Haertel (1980) reported, density values within the cavernous hemangioma correspond to those in major blood vessels (40–45 HU). The lesion has no characteristic pattern in precontrast studies. Maximum contrast enhancement in a gradually widening ring figure in the periphery of the lesion is found between 22 and 32 s, in the portal phase, while the early arterial phase is characterized by an intense but irregular increase in density values in the periphery of the hemangioma (Fig. 36). There is no increase in density values in the center of the lesion within the first 30 s, while enhancement gradually increases in the center and decreases in the periphery up to 60 s. There was no apparent relationship between

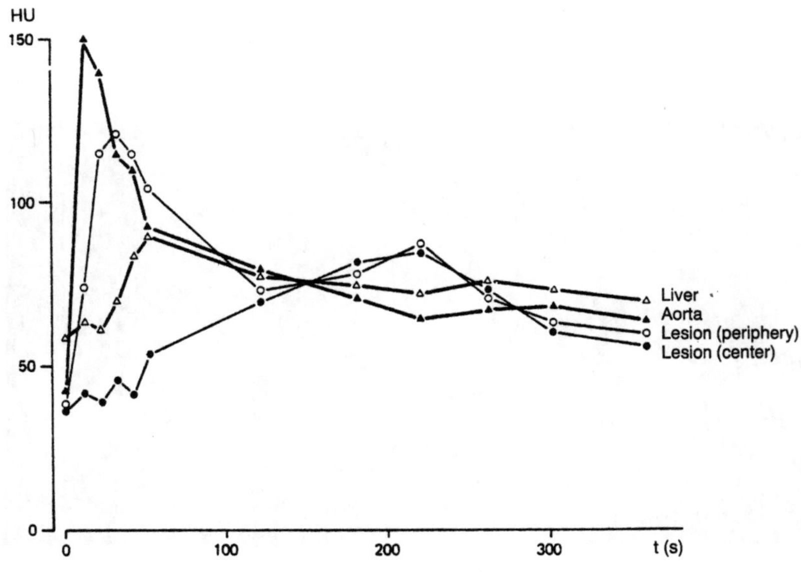

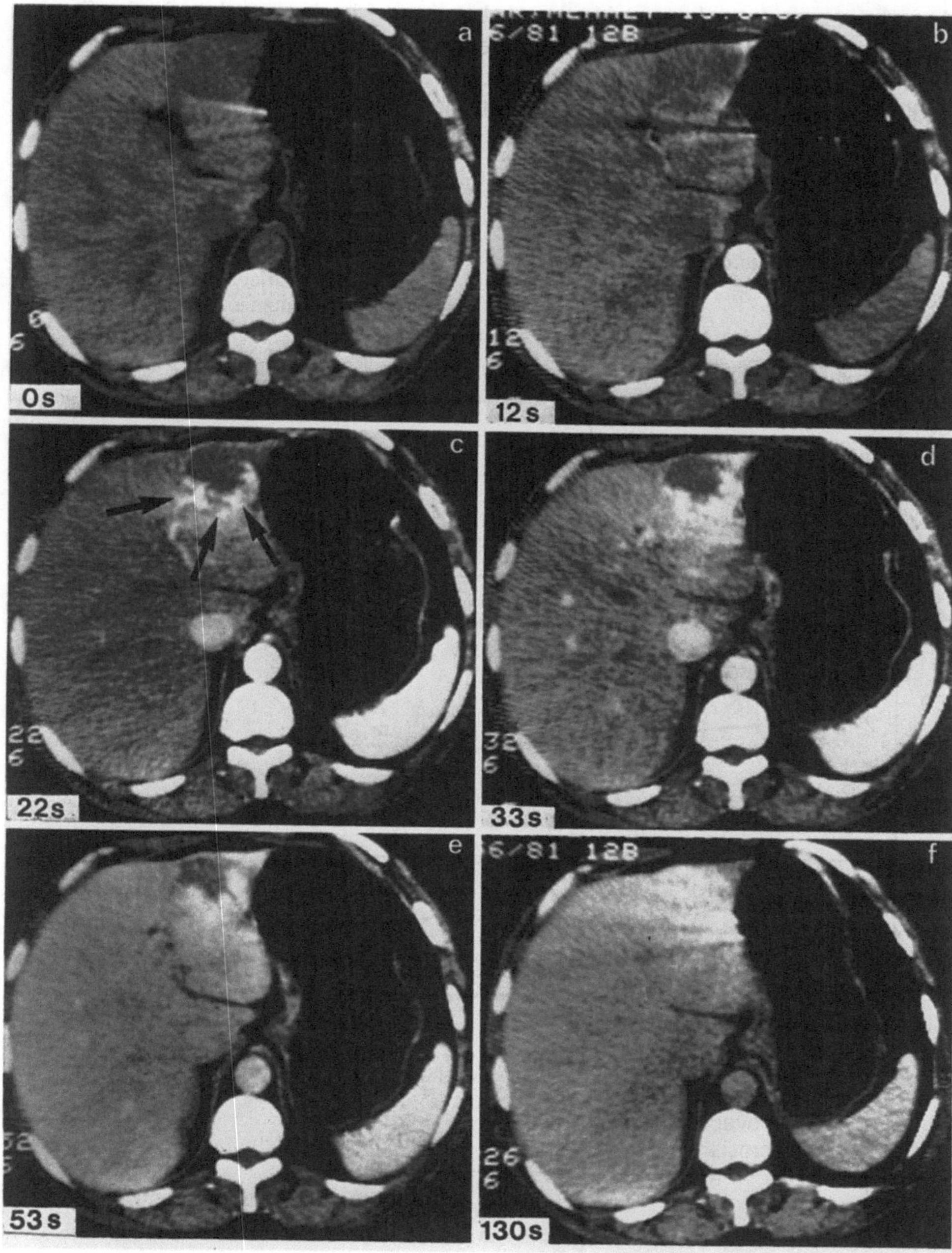

Fig. 35 a–g. Cavernous hemangioma (M. S., 44 years). Serial CT studies at 0, 12, 22, 32, 53, and 130 s. The plain scan demonstrates a hypodense zone in the left lobe of the liver. Contrast administration results in a border of contrast enhancement *(arrows)* which extends to the center of the lesion. **g** Time-density curve size of the cavernous hemangioma and duration of isodense values in the five cases of our series. In some studies hypodense zones were found to persist within the lesion after administration of a contrast agent. Haertel interpreted these findings as evidence of fibrotic obliteration following thrombosis. The same author also reported slightly hyperdense values within the hemangioma during the isodense phase.

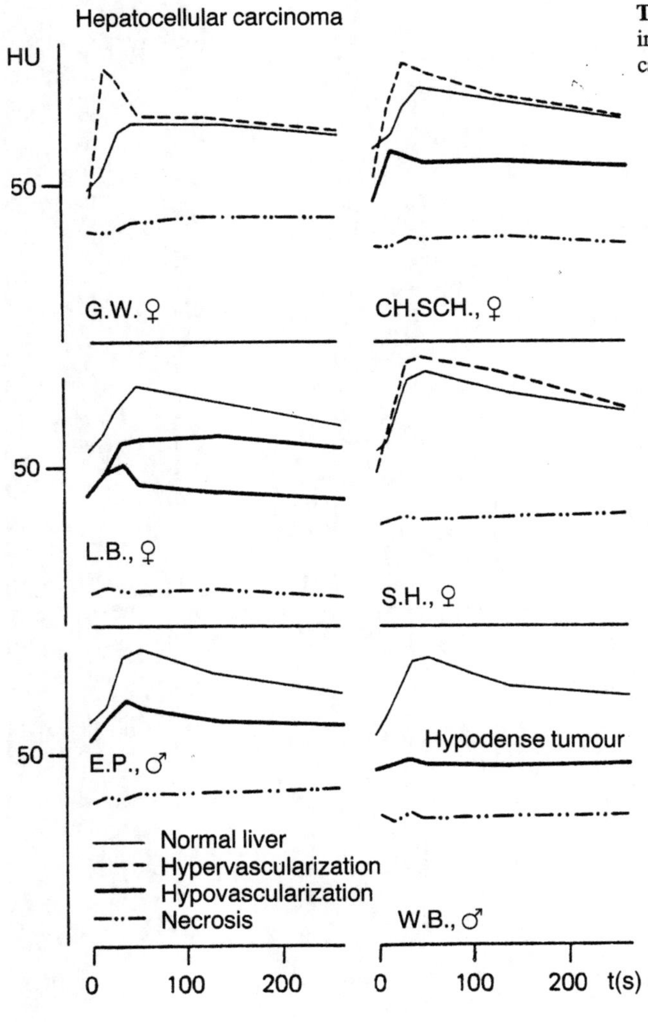

Table 2. Time-density relations in a variety of hepatocellular carcinomas

Fig. 36a–f. Cavernous hemangioma at the porta hepatis in a case of fatty degeneration of the liver ▶ (W.H., 58 years). **a** The tumor appears as a hyperdense zone which is well delineated against liver tissue with reduced attenuation values. **b** Demonstration of a few small zones of contrast enhancement at the periphery of the tumor at 12 s. **c** Demonstration of dilatation and displacement of the portal vessels in the periphery of the tumor at 22 s. **d, e** Gradual contrast enhancement from the periphery to the center of the tumor, which demonstrated homogeneous contrast enhancement at 600 s **(f)**

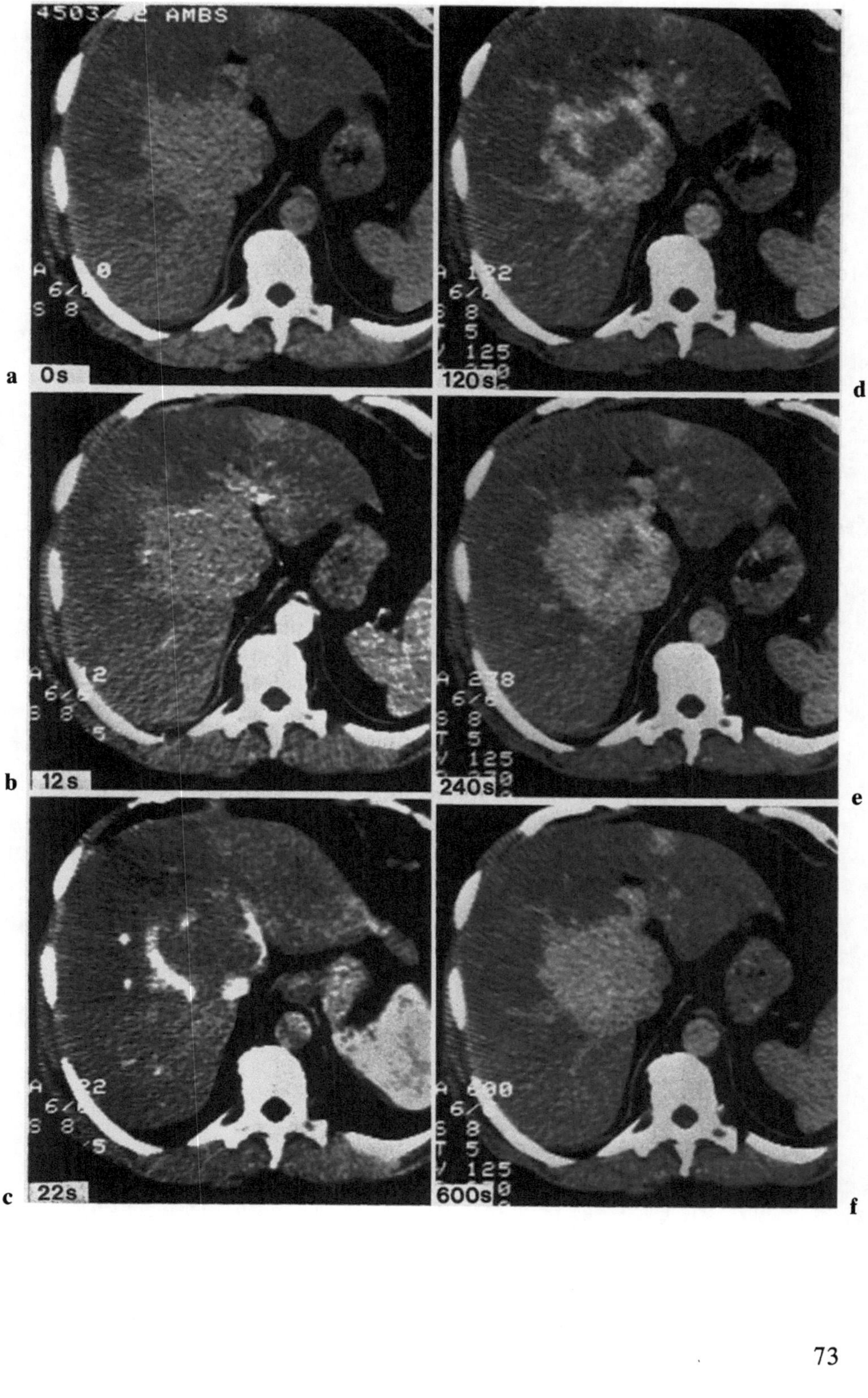
4503/82 AMBS
a
0s
b
12s
c
22s
d
120s
e
240s
f
600s

Intrahepatic abscess. The abscess appears as a hypodense zone with attenuation values approximately 30–40 HU lower than surrounding normal liver tissue in the plain scan, depending on the age of the abscess. The periphery of the lesion has somewhat higher density values than the center, with the result that the abscess is less sharply delineated than a hepatic cyst against normal liver tissue.

At 12–60 s after administration of contrast material there is a sharply delineated ring of contrast enhancement in the periphery of the lesion, which is set off from normal liver tissue by a hypodense border (Fig. 37) with the same density as normal liver tissue at 60 s; this gives the impression that the abscess decreases in size after administration of contrast material. The ring of enhancement which appears between 12 and 60 s develops in granulation tissue.

6.5.2.3 Miscellaneous Liver Lesions

Hepatic cysts are the second most common circumscribed hepatic lesions, second only to metastases. They demonstrate low density values equivalent to water as well as clearly defined borders within normal liver tissue, which allows considerable diagnostic accuracy in the plain CT scan. Administration of a contrast agent results in an increased density gradient between the cystic lesion and surrounding liver tissue. *Echinococcus cysts* often demonstrate a hyperdense ring of enhancement visible in the early arterial and portal phases up to approximately 50 s. Septation within echinococcus cysts is more readily apparent after administration of contrast material. Partial or total calcification of the walls of the cyst is also characteristic. The hyperdense ring of contrast enhancement is found in the border of granulation tissue surrounding the cyst.

Adenomas generally demonstrate a peripheral ring of contrast enhancement most pronounced in the arterial and portal phases (Fig. 38), though contrast uptake in the center of the tumor is sometimes observed. Focal nodular hyperplasia is an important consideration in the differential diagnosis of these lesions.

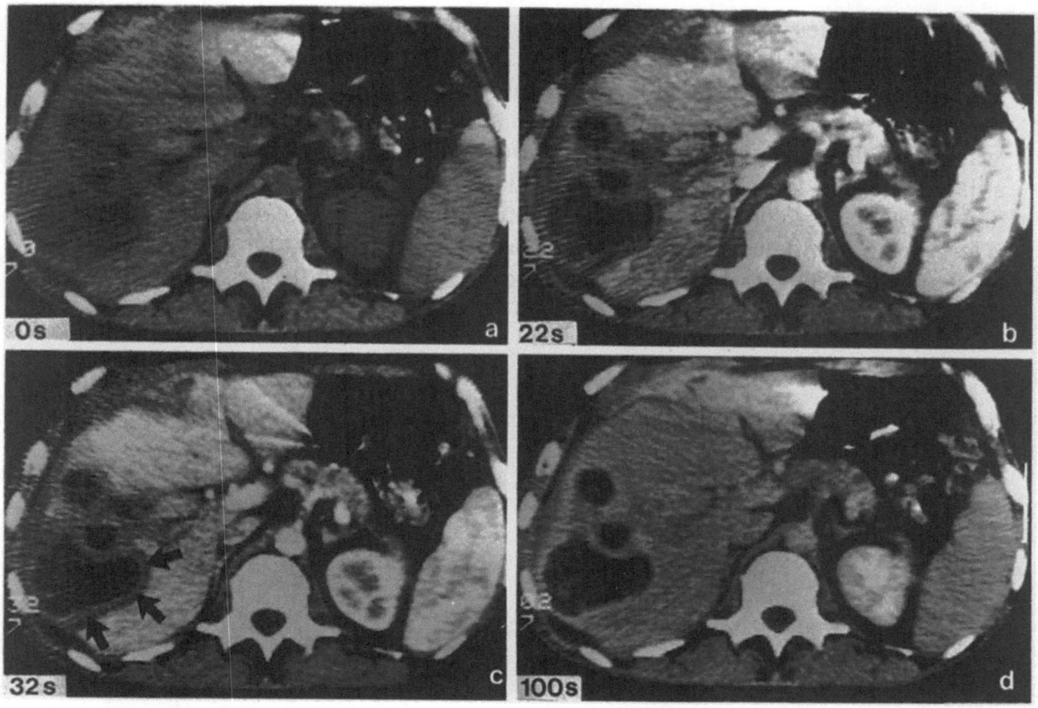

Fig. 37a–d. Pyogenic abscess in the liver (D. S., 39 years). Serial CT studies at 0, 22, 32, and 100 s demonstrate multiple hypodense zones (25–30 HU) in the right hepatic lobe. Administration of a contrast agent results in demonstration of sharply delineated rings of contrast enhancement in the periphery of the lesions *(arrows)*

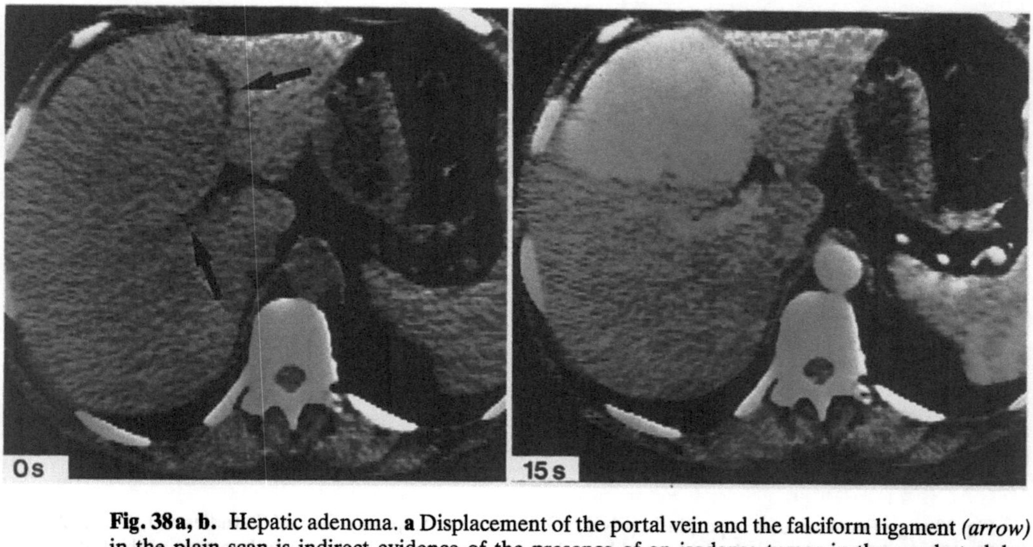

Fig. 38a, b. Hepatic adenoma. **a** Displacement of the portal vein and the falciform ligament *(arrow)* in the plain scan is indirect evidence of the presence of an isodense tumor in the quadrate lobe. **b** Strong contrast enhancement within the tumor at 15 s followed by a rapid decrease in attenuation values. (Grabbe and Heller 1982)

Density values in *focal nodular hyperplasia* average 25 HU less than adjacent normal liver tissue in the plain scan (Fig. 39). After administration of contrast material there is a rapid homogeneous increase in density within the initially hypodense zone, with a maximum in the arterial phase between 12 and 25 s. Maximum enhancement attains values approximately 15 HU higher than those in adjacent normal liver tissue (Fig. 39). This is followed by a rapid decrease in density values, with the result that the lesion is not clearly delineated at 42 s. This is followed by a rather rapid decrease in density values, which attain their original level approximately 15 HU lower than normal surrounding liver tissue at 300 s (Fig. 39).

Fig. 39 a–g. Focal nodular hyperplasia (FNH) (G. B., female, 55 years). Serial CT studies at 0, 22, 32, 52, 180, and 300 s. A sharply delineated hypodense zone is visible in the ventral portion of the left hepatic lobe in the plain scan. Administration of a contrast agent results in a rapid increase in density values within the lesion up to 32 s *(arrows)* ▶

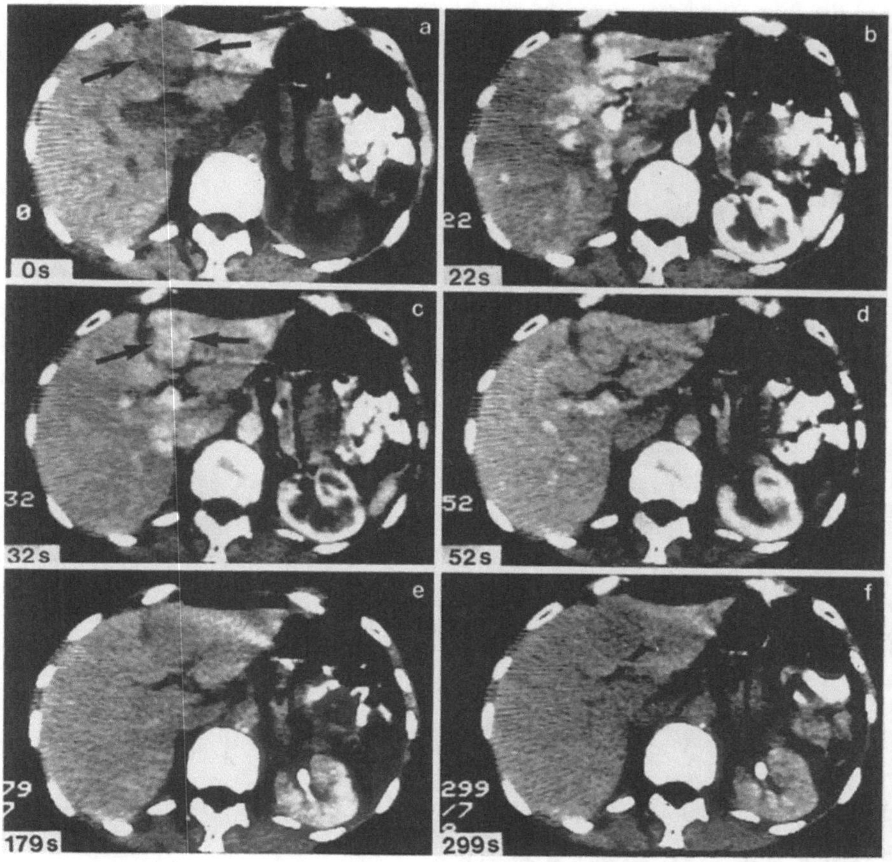
a
b
c
d
e
f
0s
22s
32s
52s
179s
299s

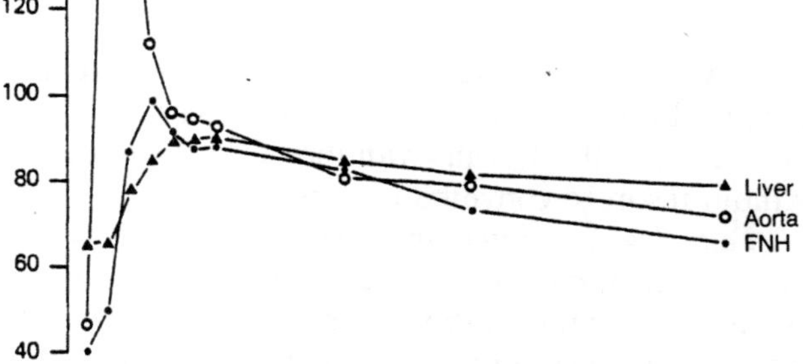
HU
180
160
140
120
100
80
60
40
0
100
200
300
t (s)
Liver
Aorta
FNH
g

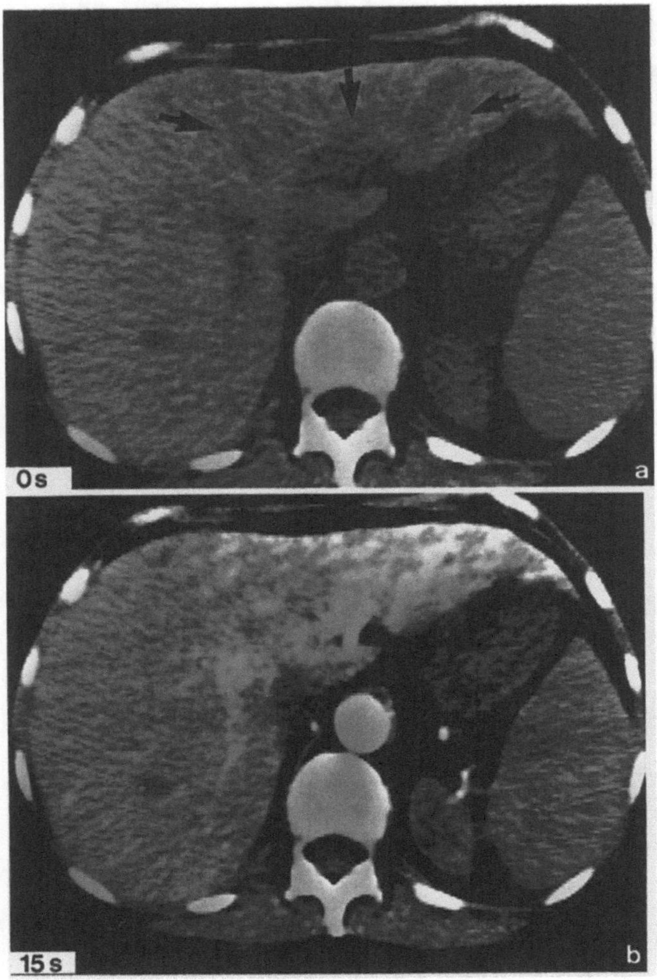

Fig. 40 a, b. Hepatic manifestation of Osler's disease. **a** Demonstration of many oval hypodense zones, especially in the left lobe, in the plain scan *(arrows)*. **b** Contrast enhancement within angiomas and AV shunts at 15 s. (Grabber and Jend 1982)

Vascular lesions such as arteriovenous fistulas, which may be found in hepatocellular carcinomas or in Osler's disease (Fig. 40), can usually be demonstrated in serial CT scans with the help of bolus injection of a contrast medium without resort to conventional angiography.

Fatty degeneration of the liver presents with hypodense values in the plain CT scan and demonstrates reduced enhancement as compared with normal liver tissue after administration of a contrast agent. There is an inverse relation between the degree of fatty degeneration and enhancement (Fig. 41), and this permits qualified conclusions as to total organ perfusion and cellular function.

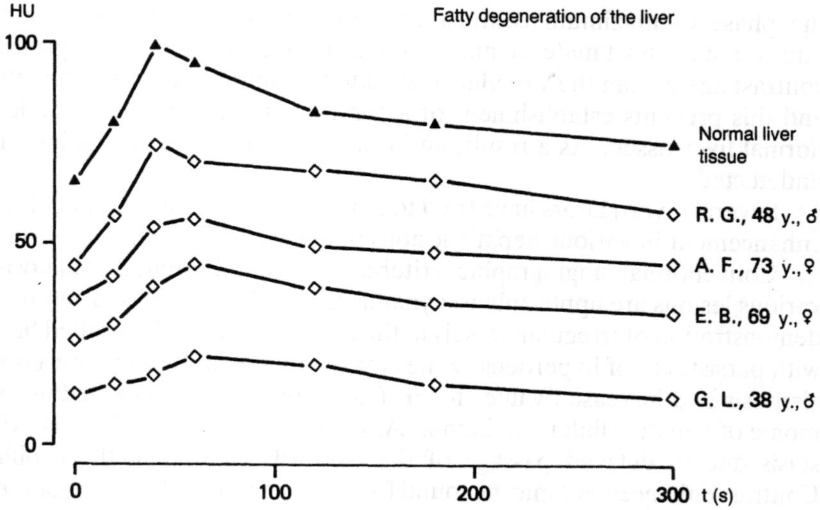

Fig. 41. Time-density curves in patients with various degrees of fatty degeneration of the liver. There is an inverse relation between contrast enhancement and degree of fatty infiltration

6.5.2.4 Critical Evaluation

The results achieved in all patients support findings reported by Rossi et al. (1981) that hepatic lesions were clearly demonstrated with dynamic CT studies. However, Moss et al. (1979) reported conflicting results, in that administration of contrast material was followed by poorer demonstration or even failure to demonstrate a lesion visible in the plain scan in 10 of 61 patients (16%). This discrepancy is explained by the fact that the studies performed by Moss did not employ the serial CT technique and bolus injection of the contrast agent. Intravenous infusion of the contrast agent as practised by Moss et al. may fail to demonstrate tumors with gradual increases in contrast values and isodense findings in later phases ("vanishing lesions"). Hepatic cysts and lipomas are easily recognized without contrast enhancement on the basis of their density values in the plain scan, and the presence of these lesions is not an indication for dynamic CT studies. The latter always resulted in better delineation of tumors and metastases as well as better definition of the extent of tumor growth and tumor volume in all other lesions under study. In some patients additional hepatic metastases which had not been visible in the plain CT scan were located in another hepatic lobe. These lesions were always smaller than 1.5 cm in diameter and were only demonstrable when the contrast gradient between the tumor and normal liver tissue was increased by administration of a contrast agent.

The principal advantage of bolus injection of contrast material with subsequent serial CT studies over conventional intravenous infusion of the contrast agent lies in the delineation of a highly vascular or avascular hepatic lesion during the phase of maximum contrast enhancement within the liver. Intravenous infusion of contrast material may result in continuously increasing passage of the contrast agent from the vascular space into the tumor and normal hepatic tissue, and this prevents establishment of a contrast gradient between the lesion and normal liver tissue. As a result, an intrahepatic space-occupying lesion may go undetected.

Several investigators have tried to define characteristic dynamics for contrast enhancement in various hepatic lesions in dynamic CT studies.

Conventional angiographic criteria for the differential diagnosis of the various lesions are applicable to dynamic CT studies. Increased vascularity with demonstration of irregular vessels in the arterial phase and so-called blood pools with persistence of hyperdense zones for several seconds in the presence of liver cirrhosis and increased values for α_1-fetoprotein can be regarded as pathognomonic of hepatocellular carcinoma. After the arterial phase there is evidence of stasis due to delayed passage of the contrast material in the capillary bed. Contrast enhancement may be found from the arterial to the portal phase in some cases of hepatocellular carcinoma. In addition to irregular hypervascular zones, CT studies may demonstrate poorly vascularized or avascular partially necrotic hypodense zones which result from obstruction of blood vessels and reduction of circulation within the tumor. Infiltration of the portal circulation also causes reduced portal blood flow with reduction of density values in some areas of the liver not directly affected by tumor.

Diagnosis of cavernous hemangioma is almost always possible with dynamic CT studies by reason of a characteristic pattern of contrast uptake in these lesions. In agreement with Haertel (1980), Freeny et al. (1979), and others, we found a broad zone of contrast enhancement at the periphery of a solitary hypodense space-occupying lesion shortly after injection, with further enhancement in the portal phase. Later in the study, movement of the contrast medium from the periphery to the center results in a gradual reduction in the size of the central hypodense zone. Haertel compared this to the action of the iris. The lesion is isodense at 3 min and becomes hypodense thereafter. Further diagnostic procedures are not necessary when this characteristic pattern of enhancement is demonstrated in the CT scan.

Older abscesses may demonstrate the same low density values as cysts and are difficult to demonstrate without the use of contrast agents. Gradual enhancement in the periphery of a hypodense lesion between 20 and 50 s after injection of the contrast medium is pathognomonic of an abscess. Density values in the peripheral ring are lower than those of adjacent liver tissue. If this ring structure, which develops in granulation tissue, is absent, then it is impossible to differentiate between abscess and cyst in the dynamic CT study.

Araki et al. (1980) proposed a classification for differentiation of intrahepatic lesions based on the contrast gradient between the tumor and normal liver tissue at defined points in time after injection of a contrast agent. Graphic representation of contrast gradients over time helps to define the moment at which a tumor can be most clearly differentiated from surrounding liver tissue. However, we believe that analysis of the degree of vascularity on the basis of absolute time-density values in normal and pathologically altered liver tissue provides clearer results and is more likely to aid in the differential diagnosis of hepatic space-occupying lesions.

6.6 Pancreas

Modern CT systems are capable of demonstrating the pancreas in nearly 100% of cases. Difficulties arise in delineating the pancreas against other retroperitoneal structures in emaciated patients with little retropancreatic fat. Changes in the size, shape, and normal limits of the pancreas are the criteria for diagnosis of pancreatic lesions in the CT scan. Circumscribed distension of the pancreas with abrupt changes in normal contours is a more reliable sign of a pancreatic space-occupying lesion than is an increase in the absolute size of the entire organ. Circumscribed distension is visible in the plain CT scan. Oral application of a contrast medium is useful in cases in which the pancreas cannot be delineated against the duodenum and other portions of the small intestine.

The shape of the pancreas is variable. The borders of the organ are usually smooth, but obese patients may demonstrate lobulated borders. Haertel et al. (1980) and Kreel et al. (1978) defined mean normal limits for the dorsoventral dimensions of the pancreas in each segment of the organ.

Ferruci et al. (1979) maintain that any increase in the size of the pancreas above 3 cm measured perpendicular to the long axis of the organ must be considered pathologic. In addition to documenting changes in the shape, size, and contours of the organ, CT studies provide density measurements which aid in the differential diagnosis of pathologic changes, especially through demonstration of pseudocysts and calcification in chronic pancreatitis. The pancreatic duct and the common bile duct are demonstrable when they exceed 5 mm in diameter. Low density values suggest the presence of edema or necrosis in acute pancreatitis. However, the fact that no density values are pathognomonic of neoplastic or inflammatory changes causes problems in differential diagnosis. Both pancreatitis and neoplasms within the pancreas may have the same density as normal pancreatic tissue, which averages 30–45 HU less than the liver.

There has been a demonstrable increase in the incidence of pancreatic carcinoma in industrial nations in recent years. Cubilla et al. (1978) reported that 3% of all patients with neoplastic disease and 5% of all patients dying of cancer in the United States had pancreatic neoplasms. Most pancreatic tumors are discovered rather late. Some 85%–90% of patients with pancreatic carcinoma demonstrate a metastasis or extension of the neoplasm beyond the borders of the organ at exploratory laparotomy. The principal role of CT lies in the detection of small resectable carcinomas less than 3 cm in diameter. Since it is often impossible to differentiate between inflammatory lesions and neoplasms in the plain scan, a number of centers have employed dynamic CT studies in an effort at discriminating between these lesions.

Bolus injection of contrast material is followed by clear demonstration of peripancreatic arteries and veins in the various phases of the CT study. Since the organ is highly vascular, maximum enhancement occurs between 15 and 25 s, and averages 20 HU higher than in the liver, with a maximum increase of approximately 50 HU as compared with the plain scan. Density values decline more rapidly than in the liver, and are approximately 30% higher than baseline at 1 min after injection of the contrast agent.

Dynamic CT studies should be performed under the following conditions:

1. Diffuse increase in the size of the pancreas and poor delineation of the organ against adjacent structures
2. Circumscribed distension of a portion of the pancreas
3. Inhomogeneous density values within the entire organ or a portion thereof

When plain CT findings demonstrate edema, hemorrhage, or necrosis within the pancreas in patients with characteristic clinical symptoms and signs of acute pancreatitis, dynamic CT studies are not indicated. The same is true of patients with extensive or circumscribed calcification and well delineated pseudocysts in cases of chronic inflammatory disease. Advanced pancreatic carcinoma with extreme distension of the organ, extension to adjacent structures, involvement of the major vessels, and demonstration of ascites or metastases in the liver and the lymph nodes obviates the need for dynamic CT studies.

6.6.1 Acute Pancreatitis

Mödder et al. (1981) and other authors have discussed the possibility of differentiating among the major stages of actue pancreatitis on the basis of serial CT studies. Pathologic–anatomic studies suggest differentiation between edema and necrosis. CT findings in acute pancreatitis are classified in three stages in accordance with clinical and pathologic–anatomic findings:

1. The acute edematous form
2. The moderately severe form with partial necrosis
3. The severe form with partial necrosis or hemorrhage

1. *Acute edematous pancreatitis (stage 1).* There is a slight to moderate increase in the volume of the entire organ in this stage of the disease, and the borders of the pancreas are usually slightly indistinct. Density values are usually normal in the plain CT scan, though there may be a decrease in attentuation values at the limits of the organ. Intravenous administration of a contrast agent is followed by rapid enhancement in the central portions of the gland from 10 to 25 s. The edematous border of the organ takes up less contrast material and is clearly delineated from the rest of the pancreatic tissue (Fig. 42, time-density curve: first row).

2. *Moderately severe acute pancreatitis with partial necrosis (stage 2).* In this stage of the disease there is a clear increase in the volume of the entire organ. Density values in the plain scan are often inhomogeneous, and it is not possible to differentiate between normal pancreatic tissue, edema, and necrosis. Bolus injection of a contrast agent results in contrast enhancement in normal pancreatic

Fig. 42. Time-density curves in patients with acute pancreatitis

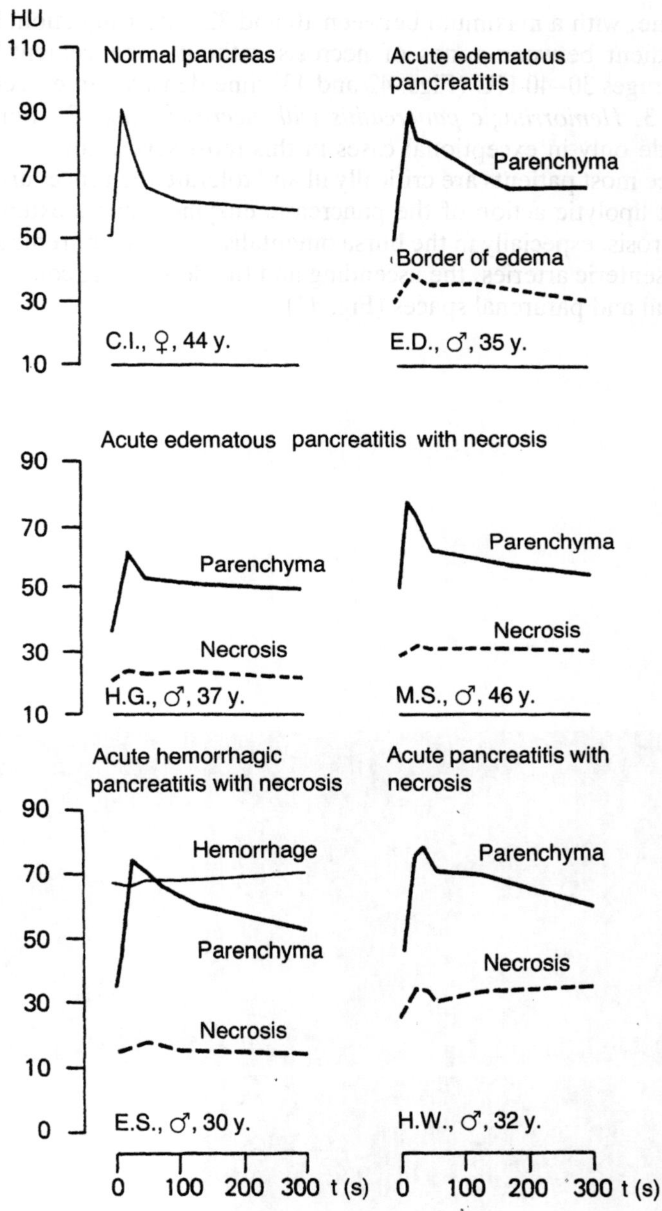

tissue, with a maximum between 10 and 32 s after injection. The mean contrast gradient between zones of necrosis without enhancement and normal tissue averages 30–40 HU (Figs. 42 and 43, time-density curves: second row).

3. *Hemorrhagic pancreatitis with necrosis (stage 3).* Serial CT studies are made only in exceptional cases in this most severe form of acute pancreatitis, since most patients are critically ill and tolerate the procedure badly. Proteolytic and lipolytic action of the pancreatic enzymes causes extensive peripancreatic necrosis, especially in the bursa omentalis, in the subphrenic space and along the mesenteric arteries, the ascending and the descending colon, and in the hepato-renal and pararenal spaces (Fig. 44).

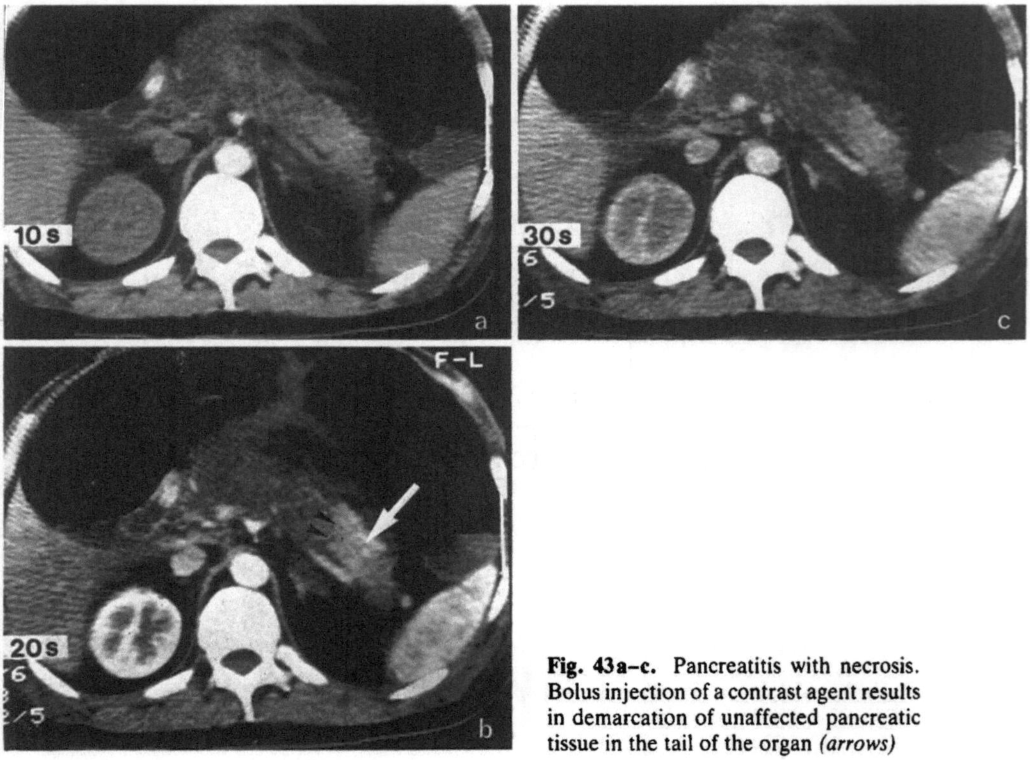

Fig. 43a–c. Pancreatitis with necrosis. Bolus injection of a contrast agent results in demarcation of unaffected pancreatic tissue in the tail of the organ *(arrows)*

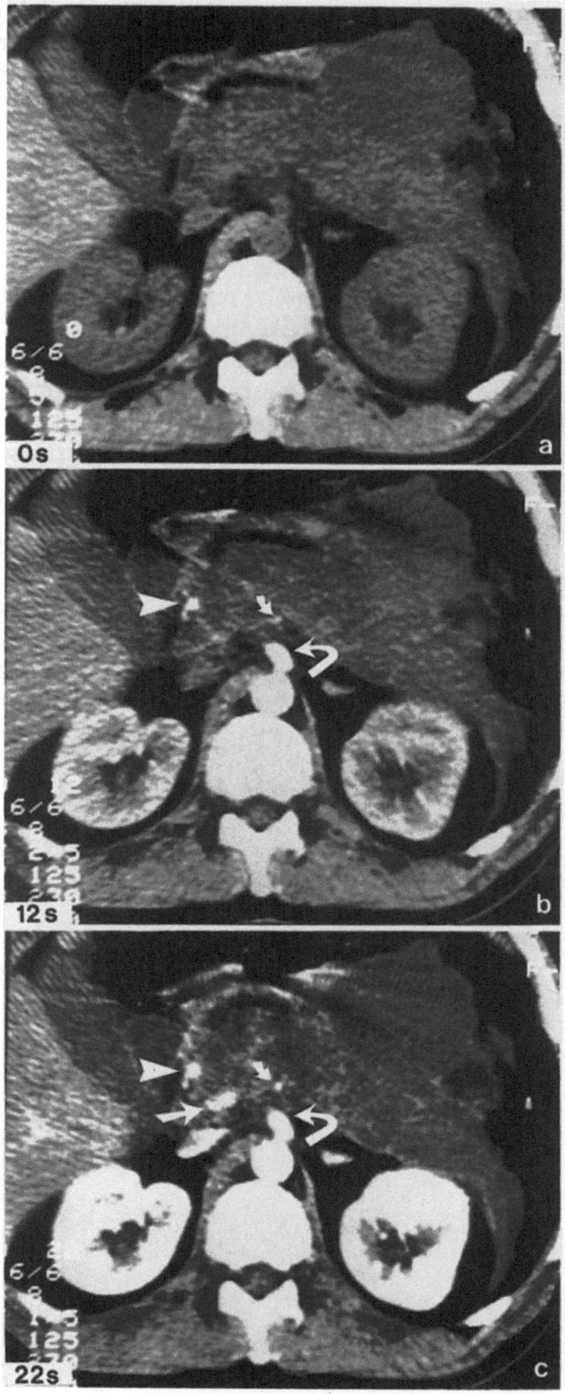

Fig. 44a–c. Severe acute pancreatitis with necrosis. There is no evidence of normal tissue after administration of a contrast agent. The following blood vessels are demonstrated: gastroduodenal artery (>), pancreaticoduodenal artery (↲), superior mesenteric artery (↶), and inferior mesenteric vein (↗)

Acute hemorrhage is readily identified and differentiated from exudates and necrosis as a result of high density values before contrast administration (Fig. 45). Dynamic CT studies are usually unnecessary in cases of severe necrotizing pancreatitis, since hemorrhage is demonstrable without the help of contrast material (Fig. 42, time-density curves: third row).

6.6.2 Chronic Pancreatitis

Pathologic–anatomic studies reveal that chronic inflammation of the pancreas is accompanied by connective tissue organization and perilobular fibrosis, and by circumscribed enlargement of the organ and development of pseudocysts in some cases. Atrophy and extensive calcification may appear in late stages of the disease. Circumscribed enlargement in chronic pancreatitis cannot be differentiated from pancreatic carcinoma if characteristic secondary signs of the neoplasm are absent.

Circumscribed enlargement of the head of the pancreas is often found in chronic pancreatitis. Cases in which atrophy of the organ is demonstrated do not require dynamic CT studies.

Serial CT studies are usually made to exclude the presence of pancreatic carcinoma. For this reason we employ dynamic CT studies only when diffuse or circumscribed enlargement of the pancreas is accompanied by nodular irregularities in the organ. Density values in the plain CT scan are similar to those in normal pancreatic tissue.

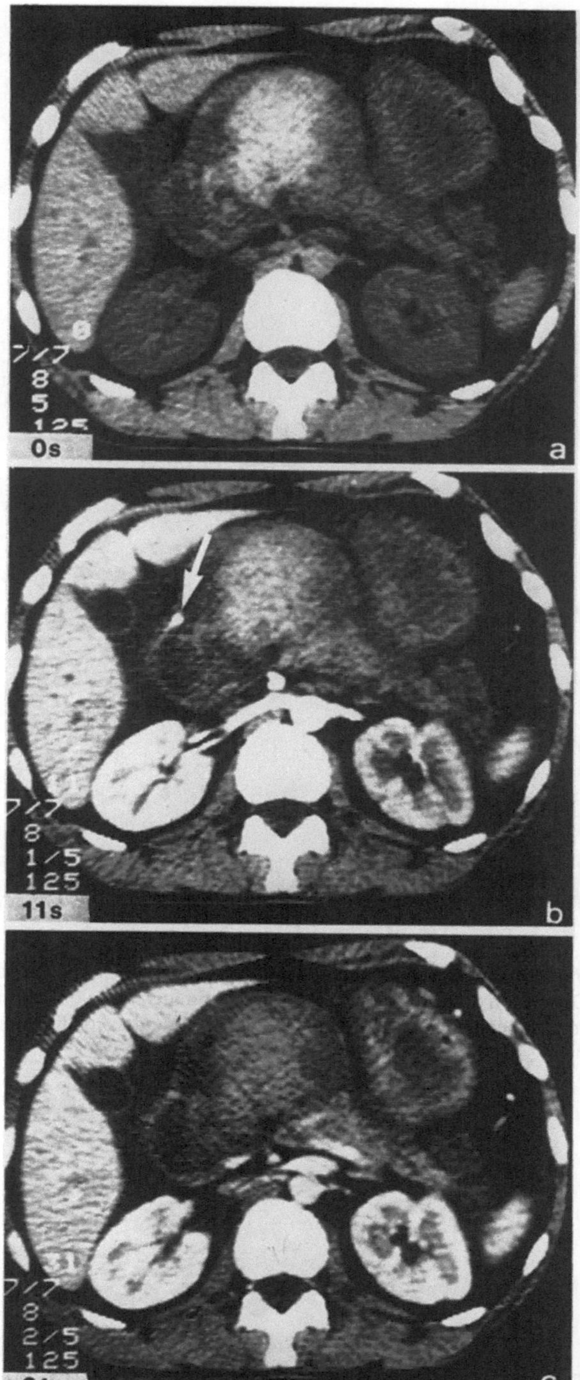

Fig. 45a–c. Acute hemorrhagic pancreatitis with necrosis (E. S., 30 years). Serial CT studies at 0, 11, and 31 s demonstrate extensive necrosis in the pancreas with penetration of the bursa omentalis. A hyperdense zone represents recent massive hemorrhage. Displacement and dilatation of the gastroduodenal artery *(arrow)*

a, b

c, d

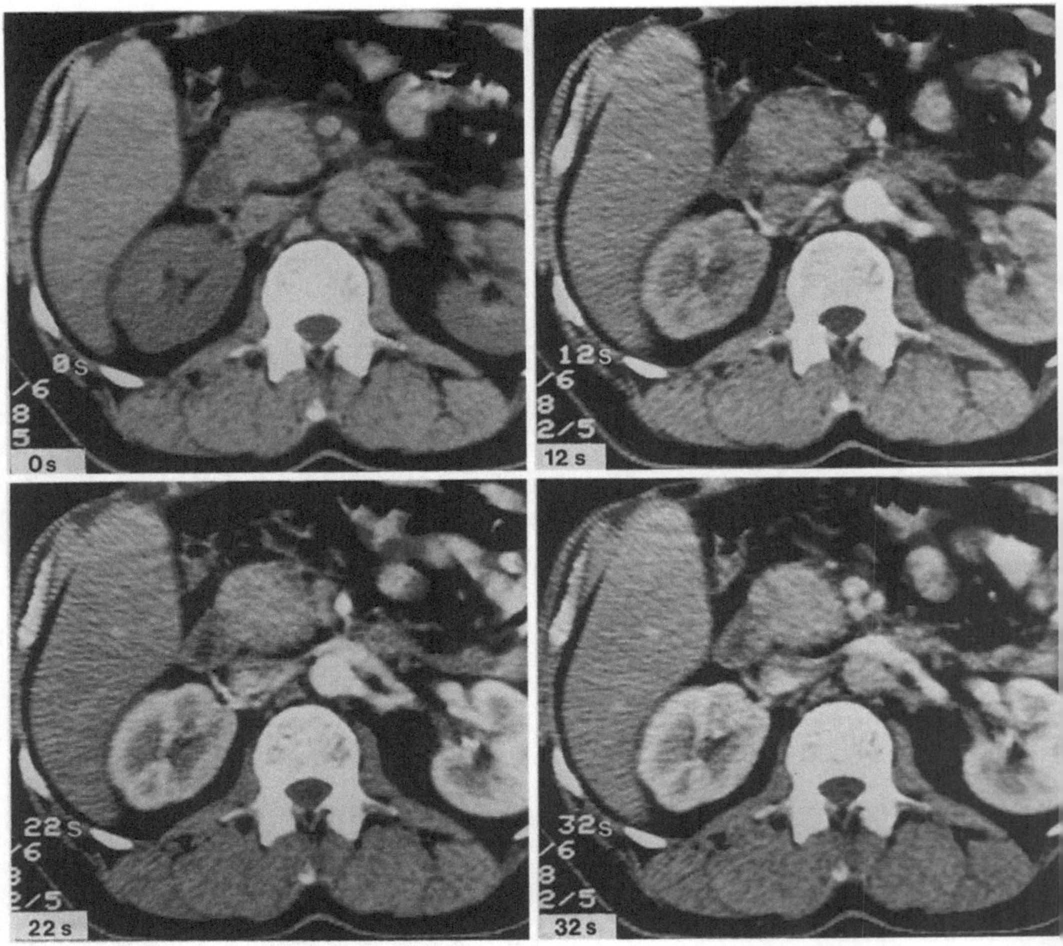

Fig. 46a–d. Chronic pancreatitis (H. S., male, 40 years). Serial CT studies at 0, 12, 22, and 32 s. Distension of the head of the pancreas. Administration of a contrast agent is followed by delayed and reduced enhancement in the pancreas (cf. time-density diagram, Fig. 47, second row left)

Maximum density values are usually lower than normal during the perfusion phase in most cases of chronic pancreatitis, especially when sclerosis is present (Fig. 46). Density values average 10–20 HU, and maximum enhancement is delayed to 40–50 s after administration of the contrast agent, as compared with 10–25 s in normal tissue (Figs. 46, 47).

Fig. 47. Time-density curves in patients with chronic pancreatitis

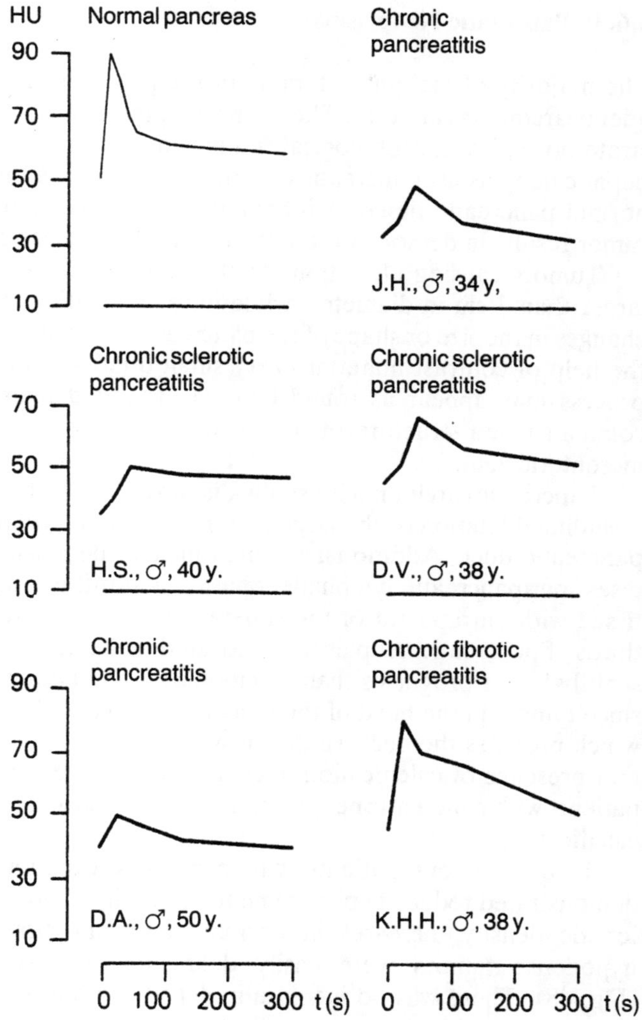

6.6.3 Pancreatic Neoplasms

The majority of malignant tumors in the pancreas are adenocarcinomas; cystadenocarcinomas are rare. The adenocarcinomas are solid tumors which demonstrate no typical morphological findings or density values in CT scans. Unlike hepatic neoplasms, pancreatic carcinomas often have the same density values as normal pancreatic tissue or inflammatory lesions. Extensive necrosis within a tumor results in demonstration of irregular hypodense zones.

Tumors causing alterations in the contours of the pancreas are generally larger than 3 cm in diameter, while intrapancreatic tumors not associated with changes in the size or shape of the pancreas are usually not demonstrable without the help of contrast material. Very small tumors in the region of the uncinate process may appear as round or oval distended figures which obliterate the comma-shaped structure of the uncinate process located behind the superior mesenteric vein.

Pancreatic carcinoma is usually diagnosed on the basis of secondary changes, including dilatation of the large extrahepatic and intrahepatic bile ducts and the pancreatic duct. Additional features include demonstration of hepatic metastases, peripancreatic lymphadenopathy, and diffuse infiltration of surrounding tissue with entrapment of the superior mesenteric artery. Approximately two-thirds of pancreatic neoplasms are located in the head of the pancreas and have a slightly better prognosis than carcinomas in the body and the tail of the organ, since tumors in the head of the pancreas may cause biliary obstruction early on, which provides the decisive diagnostic sign. Ferruci et al. (1979) demonstrated that presence of calcification does not exclude pancreatic carcinoma, as 4% of patients with pancreatic neoplasms in this series also had chronic pancreatitis with calcification.

In 69% of our patients with pancreatic carcinoma, dynamic CT studies demonstrated reduced enhancement within the tumor as compared with characteristic density increases in normal pancreatic tissue, with the result that hypodense tumors were easily delineated against adjacent normal tissue (Fig. 48). There was no increase in density within pancreatic neoplasms in the early stages, while normal pancreatic tissue demonstrated a typical increase in density values.

Fig. 48. Time-density curves in patients with carcinoma of the pancreas

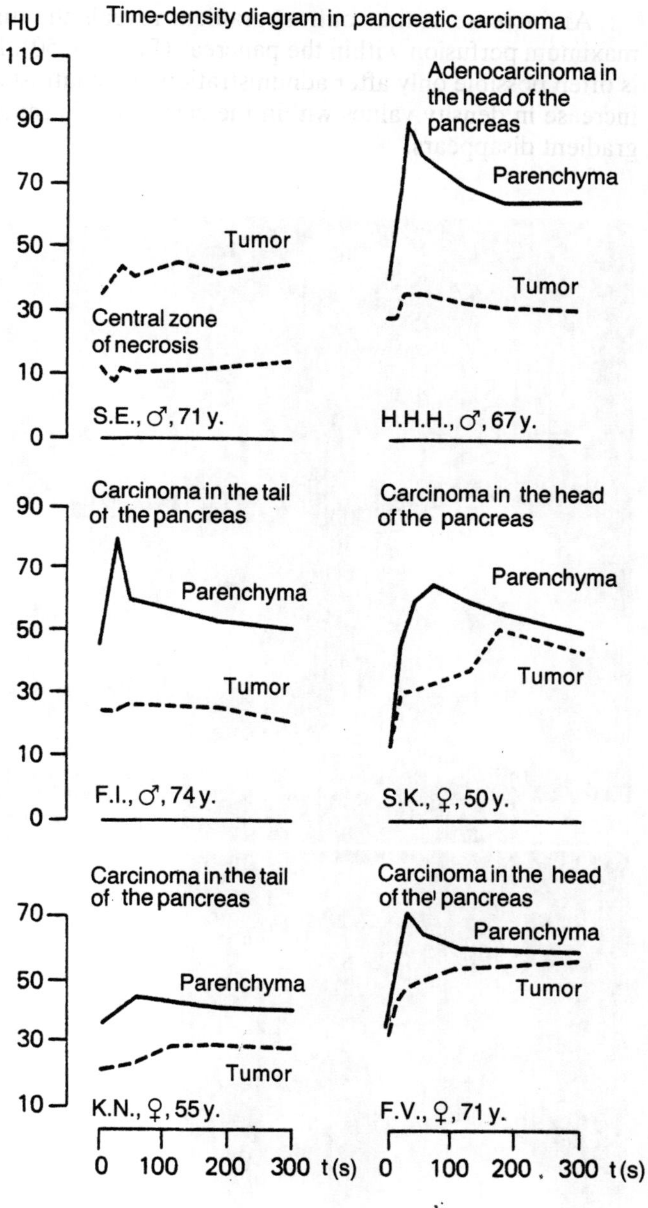

An increase in the contrast gradient reveals the tumor during the phase of maximum perfusion within the pancreas (Figs. 49, 50). Delineation of the tumor is often possible only after administration of a contrast agent. There is a gradual increase in density values within the carcinoma in same cases, and the contrast gradient disappears.

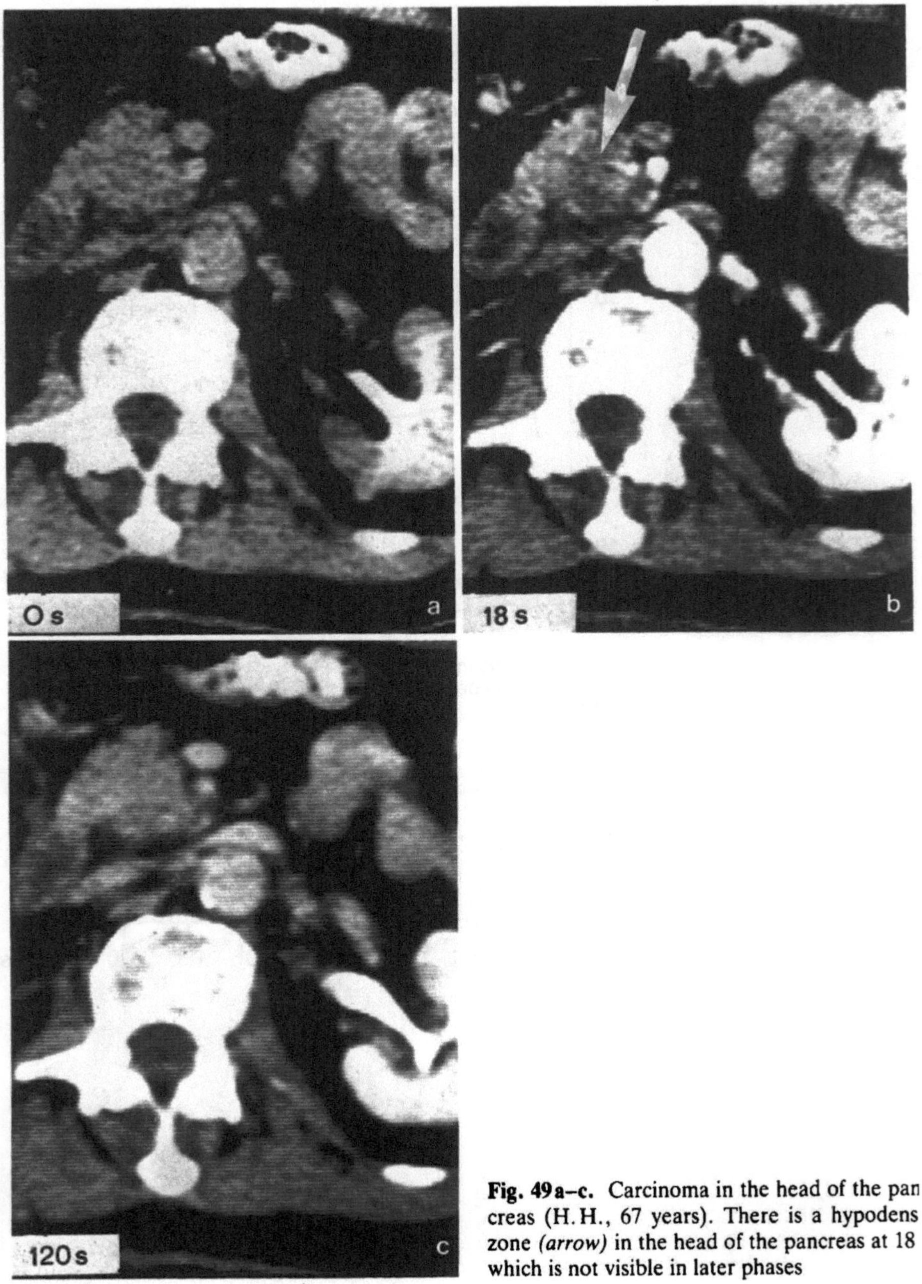

Fig. 49 a–c. Carcinoma in the head of the pan creas (H.H., 67 years). There is a hypodens zone *(arrow)* in the head of the pancreas at 18 which is not visible in later phases

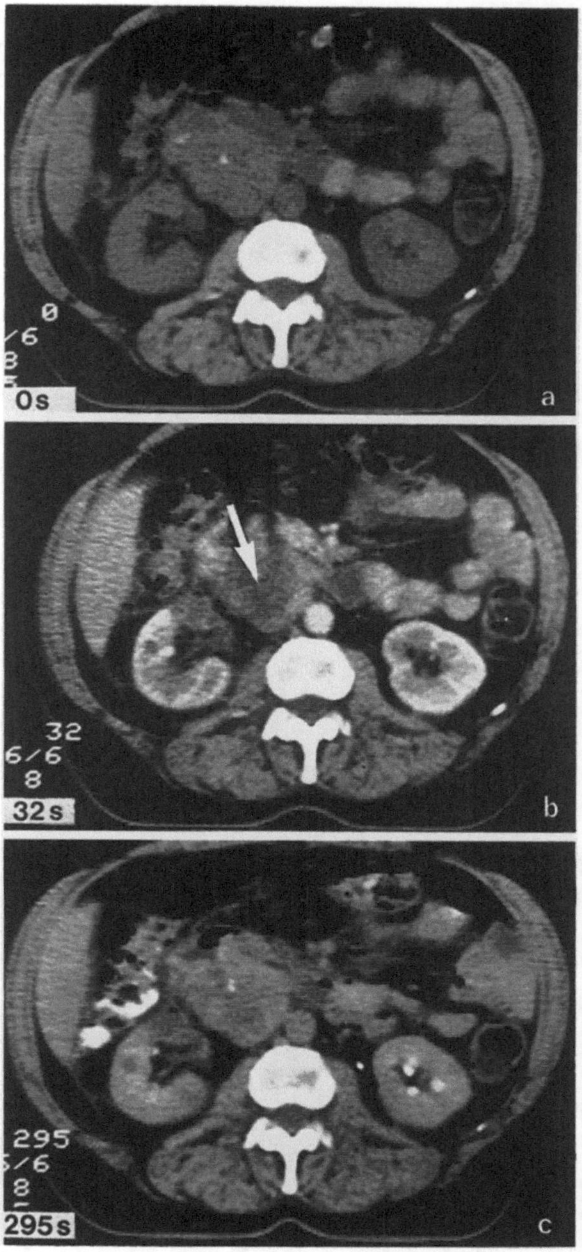

Fig. 50a–c. Leiomyosarcoma in the head of the pancreas (H.V., male, 61 years). **a** Irregular distension of the head of the pancreas with specks of calcification in the plain scan. The tumor itself is isodense. **b** After contrast enhancement the tumor appears as a hypodense zone *(arrow)*. **c** The contrast gradient is reduced at 295 s

One cystadenocarcinoma demonstrated extreme contrast uptake in a circumscribed zone as well as enhancement within the walls of the cyst (Fig. 51). In our series sensitivity was 86% with plain CT scans in cases of pancreatic carcinoma, with an increase to 95% when dynamic CT studies were performed. No false-negative findings were made.

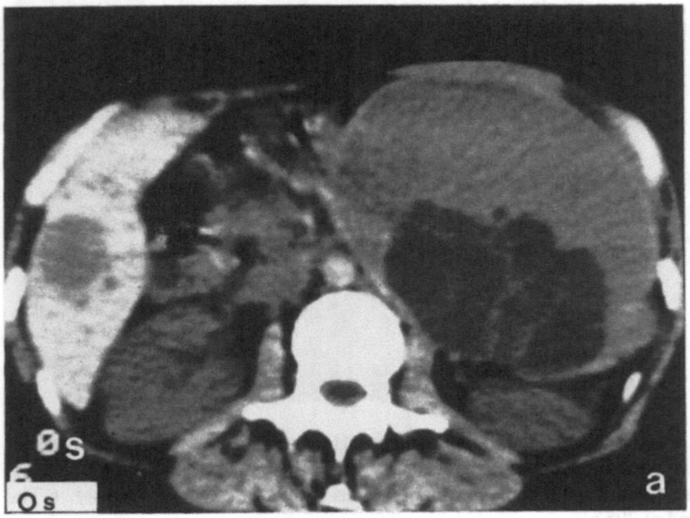

Fig. 51a–d. Carcinoma of the pancreas (B.H., female, 38 years). There is a 10×12×12 cm cystic lesion with septa originating in the tail of the pancreas. Contrast enhancement in the wall of the cyst **(b)** as well as in a circumscribed lesion *(arrow)* with a gradual decrease in attenuation values. The tumor has displaced and compressed the left kidney. There are metastases in the right hepatic lobe

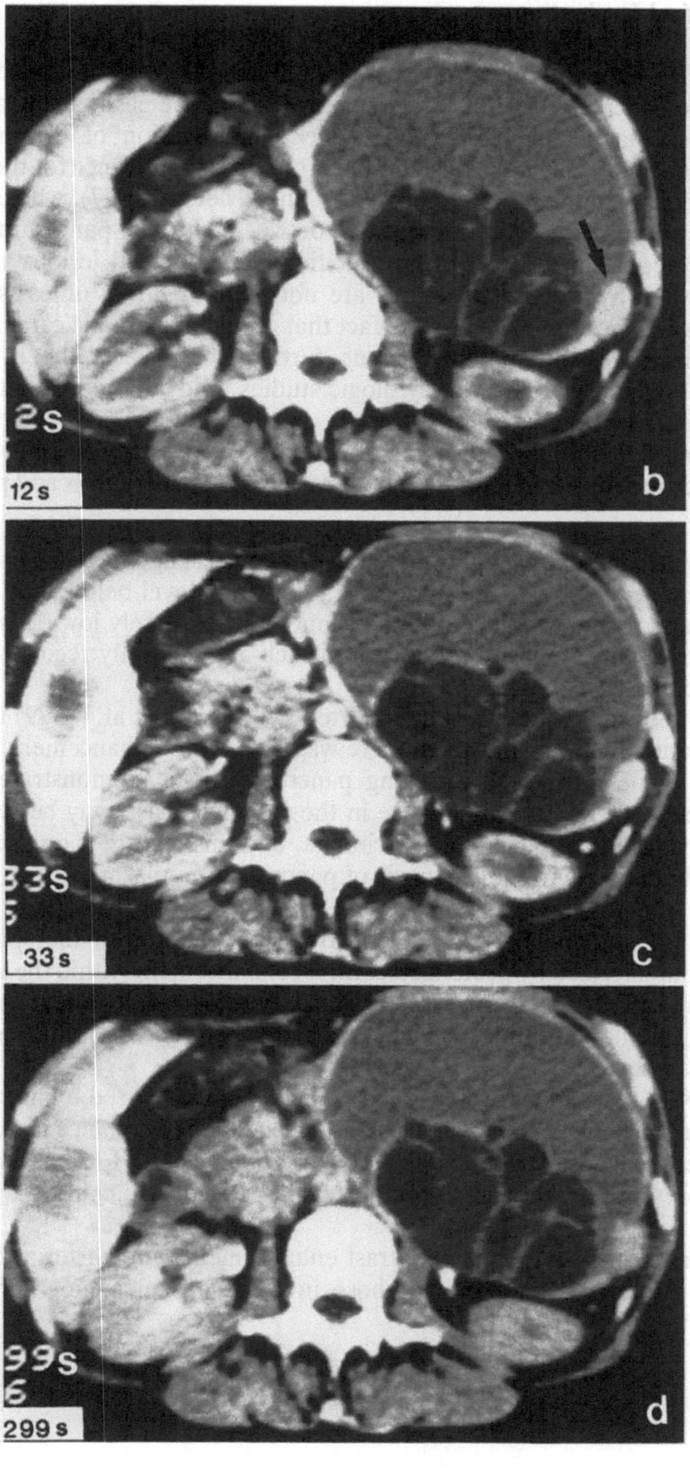
2s
12 s
b
33s
33 s
c
99s
6
299 s
d

6.6.4 Critical Evaluation

Dynamic CT studies allow diagnosis of circumscribed lesions or diffuse enlargement of the pancreas. Regions of edema or necrosis are easily delineated from normal tissue in acute pancreatitis, while demonstration of the amount of remaining normal tissue is of considerable prognostic significance for the patient.

Our findings support those reported by Sheedy et al. (1977), who concluded that it is not possible to differentiate between chronic pancreatitis and a pancreatic neoplasm in cases of noncalcified circumscribed lesions within the pancreas when hypodense structures are not demonstrated, unless secondary signs of malignancy are present. The fact that a small pancreatic carcinoma may be surrounded by inflammatory tissue further complicates the problem in differential diagnosis, and even cytologic studies following biopsy often fail to provide a definite diagnosis.

Dynamic CT studies with bolus injection of contrast material provide the following criteria for differentiation between chronic pancreatitis and pancreatic neoplasms:

1. In chronic pancreatitis, bolus injection of a contrast agent results in a delayed but homogeneous increase in density values to a level below that in normal pancreatic tissue. Absence of enhancement or extremely low density values are not found except in pseudocysts, which are generally recognized in the plain scan.
2. Our studies support the results reported by Marchal et al. (1979) in cases of pancreatic carcinoma, in which there was little or no enhancement within the lesion, while normal surrounding pancreatic tissue demonstrated normal enhancement. Failure to enhance in the vascular phase may be regarded as pathognomonic of pancreatic carcinoma, and this feature is one of the most important criteria in the diagnosis of pancreatic neoplasms.

Serial CT studies may also demonstrate compression of the splenic vein, which is characterized by prolonged contrast enhancement within the spleen and by the presence of collateral circulation. In contrast to adenocarcinomas, anaplastic carcinomas often have an extensive zone of necrosis which is visible in the plain CT scan.

Except in cases of centroblastoma, which is characterized by homogeneous contrast enhancement, pancreatic lesions which failed to enhance in dynamic CT studies were diagnosed as probable pancreatic neoplasms. However, most of our patients presented with clinical findings which raised suspicion of a pancreatic tumor.

Insulinomas show extreme contrast enhancement in the arterial phase, and these CT findings correspond to those in conventional angiographic studies (Fig. 52).

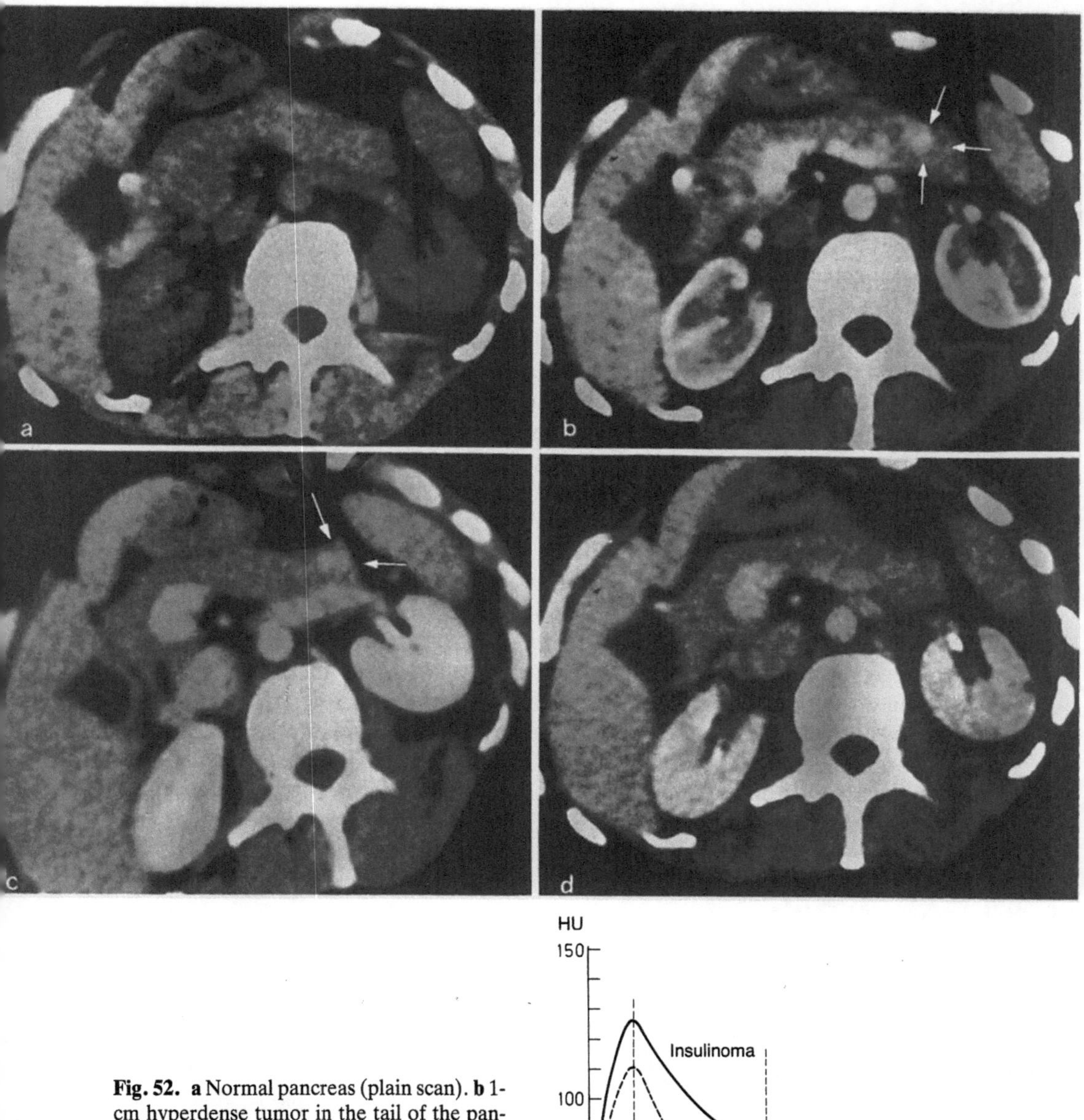

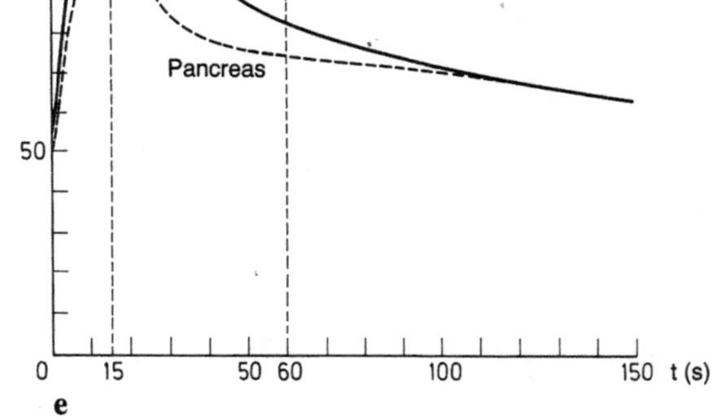

Fig. 52. **a** Normal pancreas (plain scan). **b** 1-cm hyperdense tumor in the tail of the pancreas slightly below the surface and 2 cm from the end of the organ at 15 s after contrast administration. **c** Demonstration of an insulinoma in the tail of the pancreas at 30 s with slight variation in the demonstration due to respiratory excursion; at 45 s, decrease in attenuation values within the still visible insulinoma. **d** Homogeneous density values within the pancreas at 75 s; the insulinoma is no longer apparent. **e** Time-density curve; the insulinoma is demonstrated from 15 to 60 s (Buck and Binder 1982)

6.7 Spleen

Contrast CT studies have already proved their value in the diagnosis of traumatic lesions, inflammatory disease, and tumors and in the demonstration of accessory spleens. Lesions smaller than 1 cm in diameter remain a problem, especially in the staging of lymphomas.

6.7.1 Vascular Studies

The arteries and veins at the hilum of the spleen are well demonstrated in dynamic CT studies, while the spleen itself may show homogeneous or somewhat inhomogeneous enhancement. The inhomogeneous pattern begins in the arterial phase and continues to the parenchymal phase (Fig. 53). Homogeneous contrast enhancement in splenic tissue is demonstrated at approximately 120 s. The enhancement pattern in the spleen is different from that found in other parenchymal organs, and this fact is explained by the histologic features of the splenic vessels. The sinuses of the spleen are an intermediate system of capillary spaces in the red pulp between the arterial and venous beds of the spleen. The sinuses are a three-dimensional network of vessels with varying contents. They may be packed full of red blood cells while plasma passes into the interstitial space; they may contain more white cells than red cells; or their contents may approximate the normal composition of circulating blood. Pores in the walls of the sinuses allow free exchange of corpuscular and fluid elements between the sinuses and the red pulp in both directions. The size of the openings in the walls of the sinuses varies with the contents of the sinus, and the latter functions as a type of filter and regulator of blood flow, which results in inhomogeneous contrast uptake.

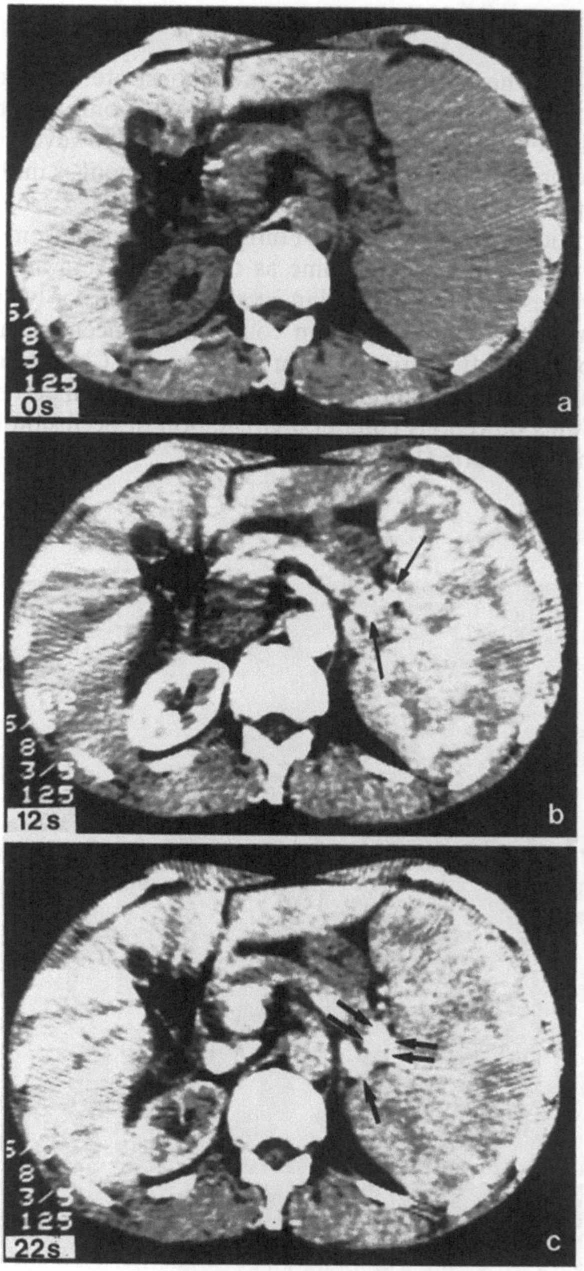

Fig. 53a–c. Splenic enlargement in hemolytic anemia (W.M., male, 49 years). **b** Contrast enhancement in the splenic artery at the hilum of the spleen *(arrows)* at 12 s; inhomogeneous density values within the spleen. **c** Demonstration of the splenic vein *(arrows)* at 22 s

6.7.2 Pathologic Findings

Since the normal spleen may demonstrate inhomogeneous contrast enhancement, dynamic CT studies often provide only slight improvement in the rate of demonstration of small tumors (Fig. 54). However, dynamic CT studies do allow improved demonstration of pathologic changes in the region of the hilum of the spleen. Accessory spleens are differentiated from enlarged lymph nodes or varicose veins by virtue of differences in enhancement. Varicose veins generally enhance at the same time as the splenic vein and demonstrate higher density values than those found in accessory spleens or lymph nodes. Accessory spleens have the same maximum contrast enhancement as the normal spleen, which permits differentiation from lymph nodes. Characteristic time-density curves also allow differentiation of dilatation or aneurysm of the splenic artery from varicose veins or venous collateral circulation in occlusion of the splenic vein or portal hypertension (Fig. 55).

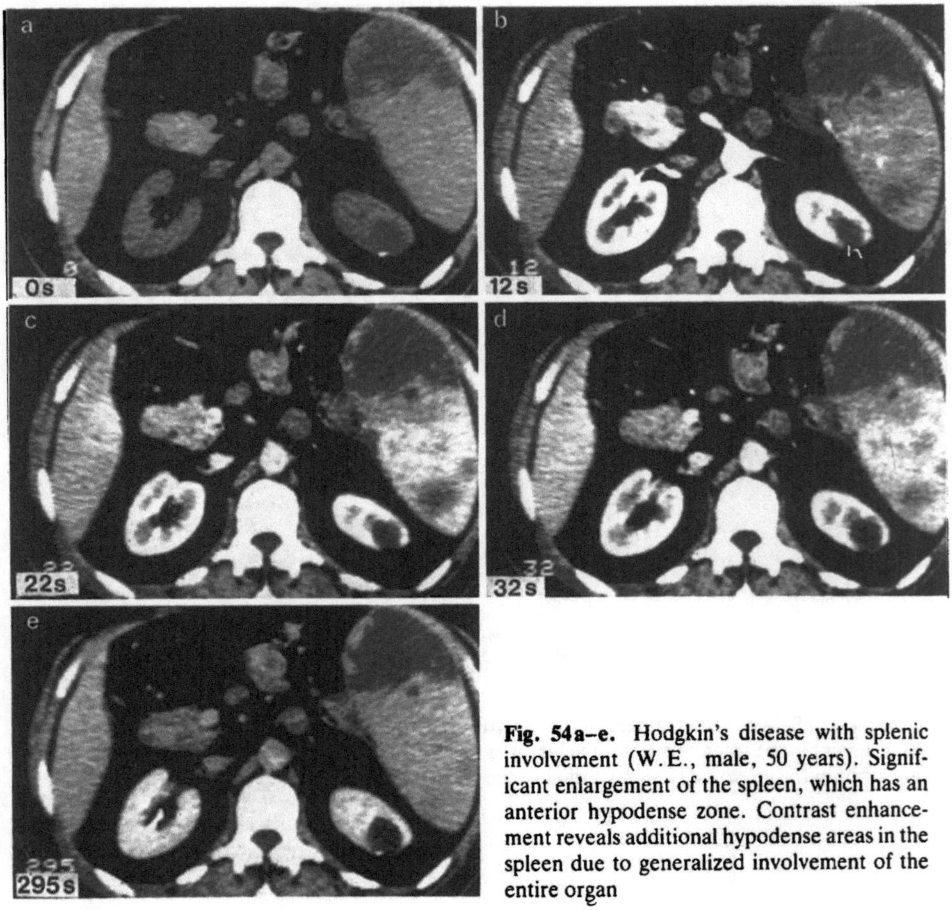

Fig. 54a–e. Hodgkin's disease with splenic involvement (W.E., male, 50 years). Significant enlargement of the spleen, which has an anterior hypodense zone. Contrast enhancement reveals additional hypodense areas in the spleen due to generalized involvement of the entire organ

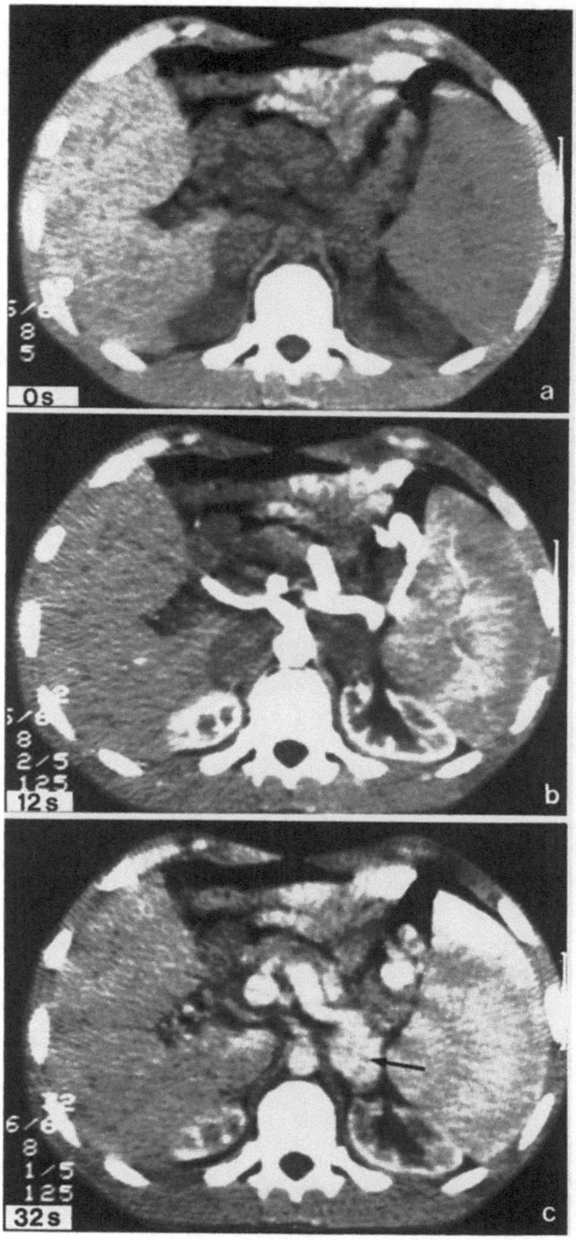

Fig. 55 a–c. Splenic enlargement secondary to congenital malformation of the splenic vessels (B. L., male, 18 years). **a** Irregular vascular structures at the hilum of the spleen in the plain CT scan. **b** Demonstration of a widened and elongated splenic artery at 12 s. **c** Demonstration of an aneurysm *(arrow)* in the splenic vein at 32 s

6.7.3 Critical Evaluation

Dynamic CT studies do not allow better demonstration of details within the spleen, since contrast enhancement is inhomogeneous in the normal organ. As a result it is hardly to be expected that scanners with better resolution will improve results in staging of lymphomas. However, use of iodinated fat emulsions such as EOE-13 does improve results. Dynamic CT studies do represent progress in the diagnosis of pathologic changes in the hilum of the spleen.

6.8 Retroperitoneal Space

6.8.1 Kidneys

The kidneys are located in the lumbar fossa and are usually well demonstrated in CT studies. The medulla and the cortex are not well differentiated in plain CT scans, though the fat in the medullary sinus is well delineated. Density values in normal renal tissue average 35 HU. Following bolus injection of a contrast agent there is significant contrast enhancement and clear demarcation of the peripheral renal cortex during the arterial phase (10–20 s), with maximum density values as high as 140 HU. After a slow decrease in enhancement in the cortex, density values increase in the medulla, and there is homogeneous enhancement in the tubular phase (60–120 s) followed by demonstration of contrast material in the renal pelvis. Demonstration of the renal vessels is usually incomplete in a single slice.

Time-density curves in normal kidneys (Fig. 56) represent the sum of three simultaneous functions – perfusion, diffusion of the contrast medium into the interstitial space, and excretion of the contrast medium into the renal pelvis and the ureters. Density values in the renal medulla increase slowly to a peak between 60 and 120 s. Comparison of the curves described for each kidney permits conclusions on renal perfusion similar to those made in scintigraphic studies.

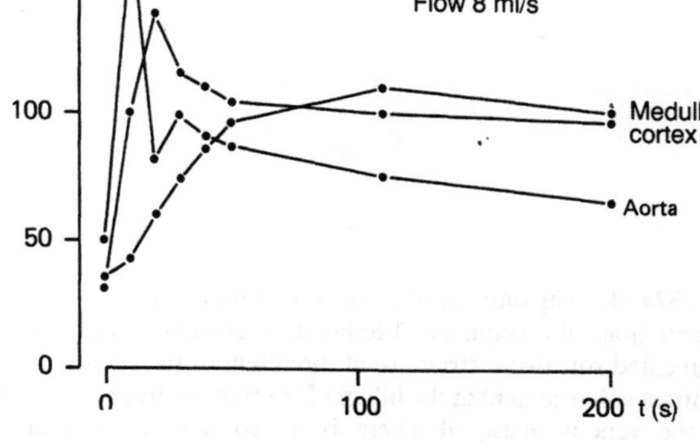

Fig. 56. Time-density curves in normal renal tissue and in the aorta

6.8.1.1 Benign Renal Tumors

Angiomyolipomas are benign mesenchymal mixed tumors composed of blood vessels, smooth muscle, connective tissue, and fat. In the plain CT scan they appear as space-occupying lesions with indistinct borders and density values representative of fat in some portions of the tumor. Demonstration of fatty tissue suggests a diagnosis of angiomyolipoma rather than adenocarcinoma. Serial CT studies allow evaluation of the vascularity of the tumor and improve delineation of the lesion (Fig. 57).

Fig. 57a–d. Angiomyolipomas in both kidneys (D. I., female, 37 years). Hypodense structures with ▶ attenuation values equivalent to fat are seen in both kidneys in the plain CT scan. There is a poorly delineated soft tissue structure at the hilum of the right kidney. **b** Irregular zones with very strong contrast enhancement at the hilum of the right kidney *(arrow)*, with **c** rapid decrease in density values in the venous phase. **d** There is no contrast enhancement in areas with attenuation values corresponding to fat *(arrows)*

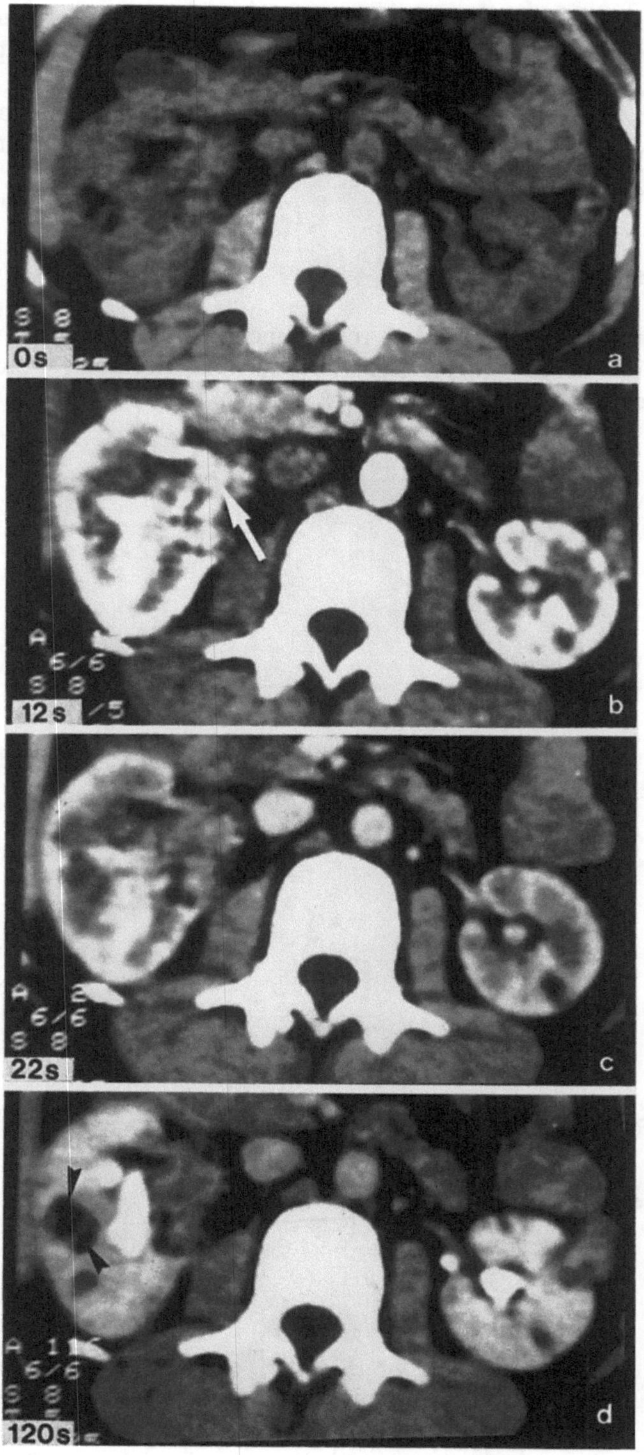
0s
a
12s
b
22s
c
120s
d

Cortical adenomas are among the most common benign renal tumors and are usually found as circumscribed space-occupying lesions near the capsule of the kidney. They are generally hyperdense in the plain CT scan and do not contain calcification. Adenomas are not highly vascular tumors, and administration of contrast material results in less enhancement within the tumor than in normal renal tissue (Fig. 58).

6.8.1.2 Renal Transplantation

Serial CT studies may be used as renal function studies in cases of evolving rejection. Time-density curves show reduced enhancement, which indicates incipient rejection (Fig. 59a, c).

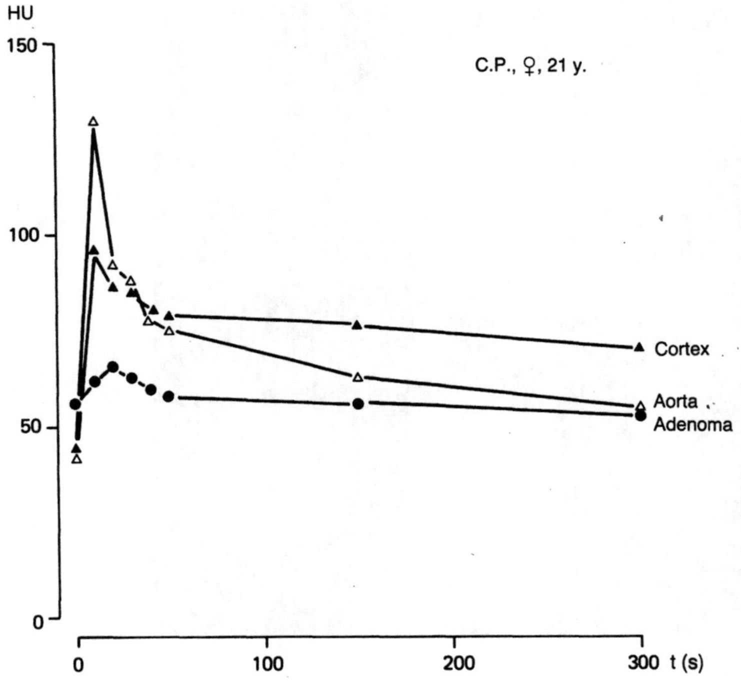

Fig. 58e

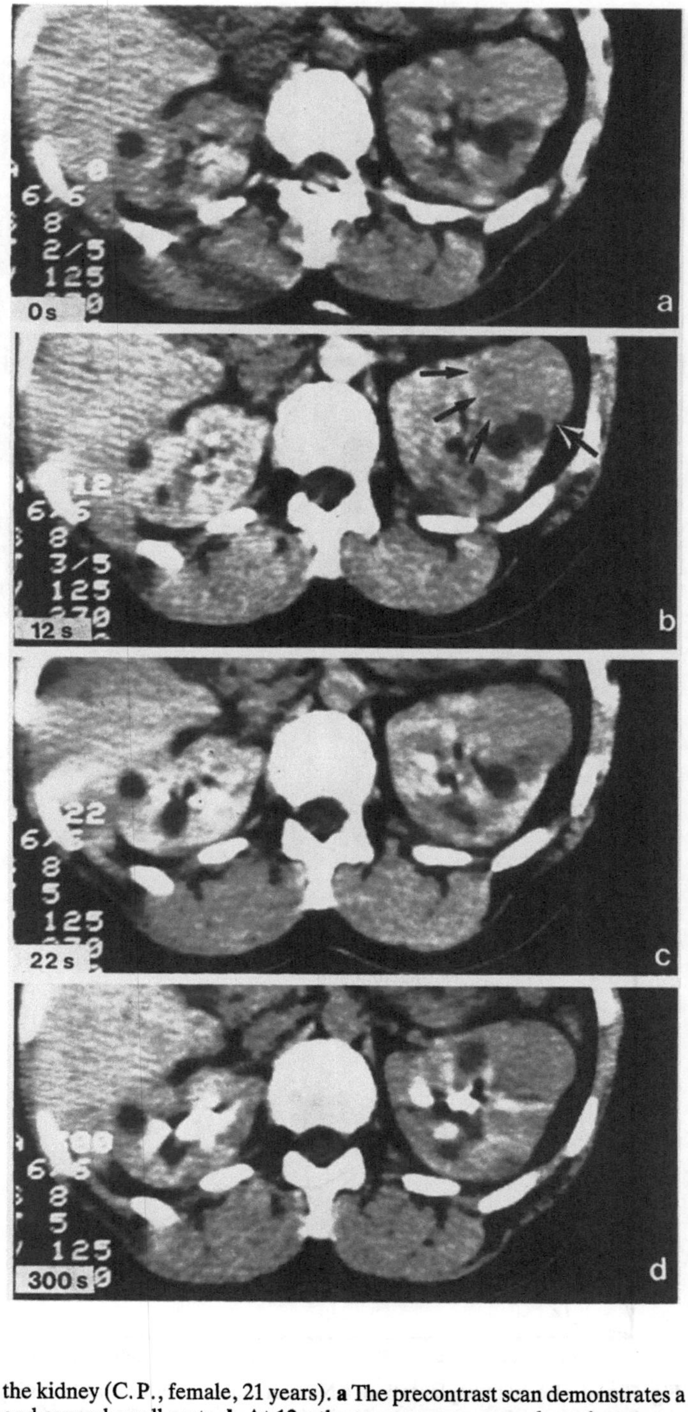

Fig. 58 a–e. Adenoma of the kidney (C. P., female, 21 years). **a** The precontrast scan demonstrates a slightly hypodense lesion and several small cysts. **b** At 12 s the tumor appears as a hypodense zone against the renal cortex and medulla *(arrows)*. There is no significant change in the contrast gradient later in the study. **e** Time-density diagram

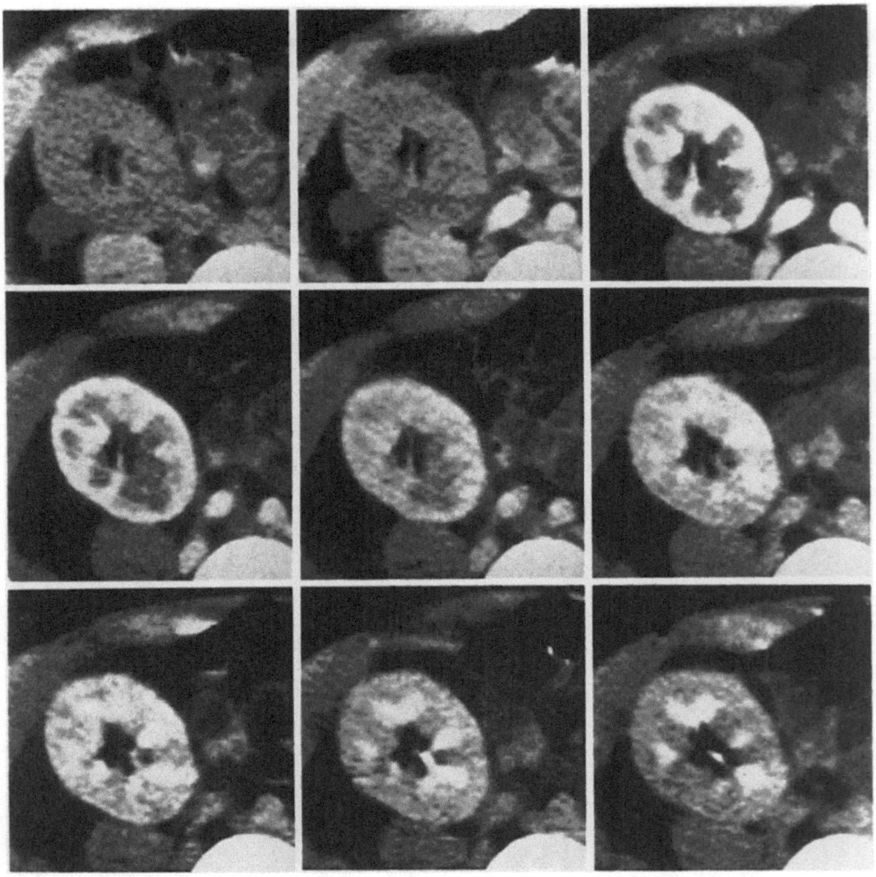

a

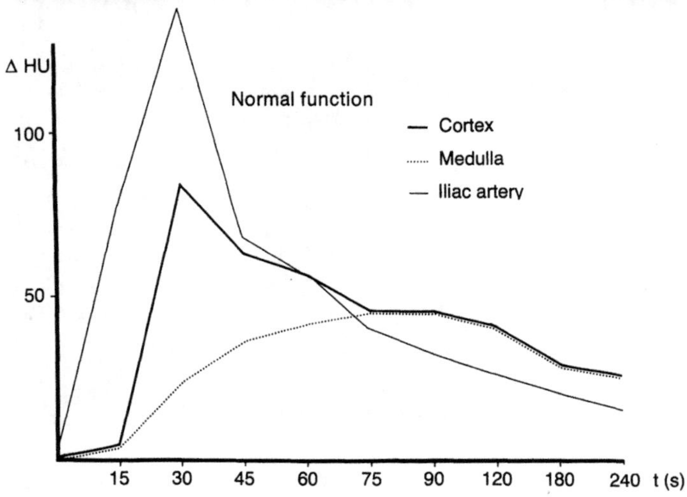

b

Fig. 59 a–d. Renal transplantation. **a** Normal function. Following bolus injection there is stasis in the tubules and strongly contrasted urine in the renal pelvis. **b** Time-density curve. **c** Pathologic function in rejection (U. A., male, 33 years). Bolus injection of a contrast agent reveals no swelling. Artifacts are found but there is no contrast in the tubules and no demonstration of urine in the renal pelvis.

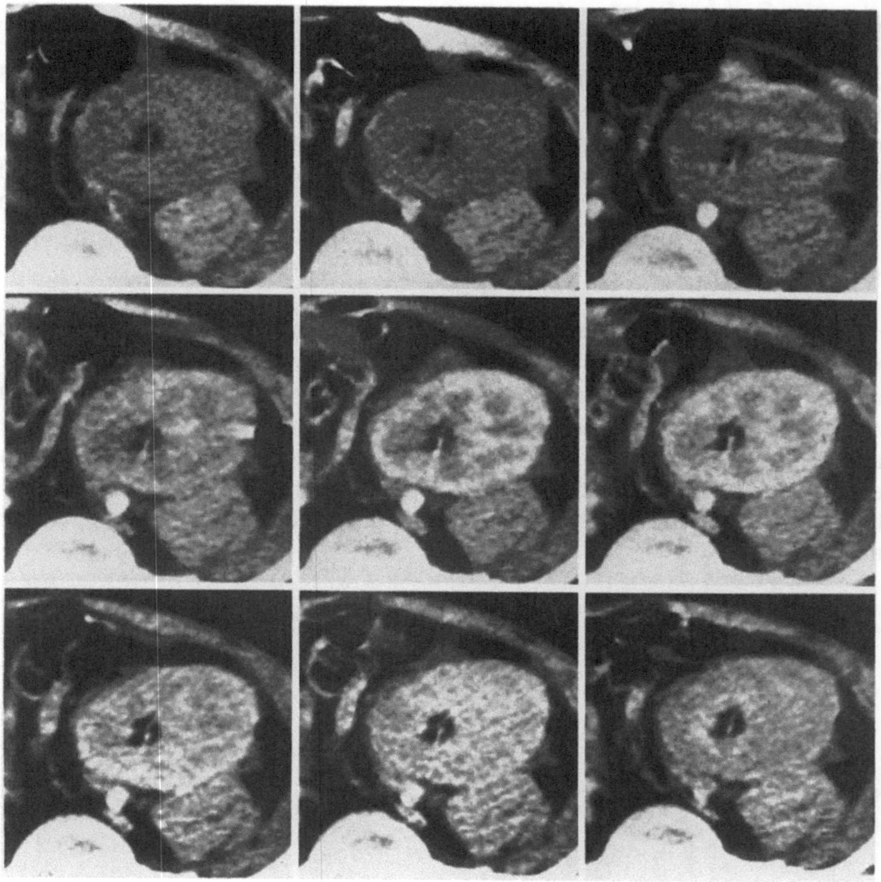

c

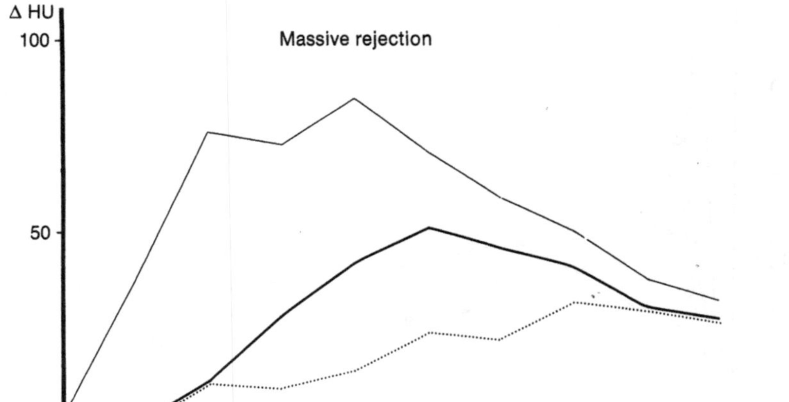

d

d Time-density curve. The cortical curve is flattened and the duration of the density gradient between the cortex and the medulla is prolonged (30–240 s). Failure to demonstrate an initial peak in the iliac artery results from the intervals chosen for the study (Treugut et al. 1981).

6.8.1.3 Renal Carcinoma

Three-quarters of all malignant renal neoplasms are adenocarcinomas; the majority demonstrate high vascularity, while approximately 10% are hypovascular and the occasional tumor is isodense. Serial CT studies demonstrate extreme enhancement in the arterial phase, which allows clear delineation of the carcinoma (Fig. 60). The contrast gradient between the tumor and normal renal tissue diminishes during the course of the study, and the lesion is less clearly defined with time.

Most adenocarcinomas have indistinct borders against normal renal tissue in the plain CT scan. The tumors present with a mixture of fatty infiltration, necrosis, and calcification. Time-density curves show pathologic hypervascularization in the tumor in the early phase of the study, which corresponds to findings with conventional angiography. The presence of arteriovenous shunts results in a rapid decrease in density values between 20 and 40 s, and the hyperdense tumor returns to its original hypodense appearance after 1 min (Fig. 60). Thrombosis of the renal vein and the vena cava may be demonstrated at the contrast maximum in the venous phase.

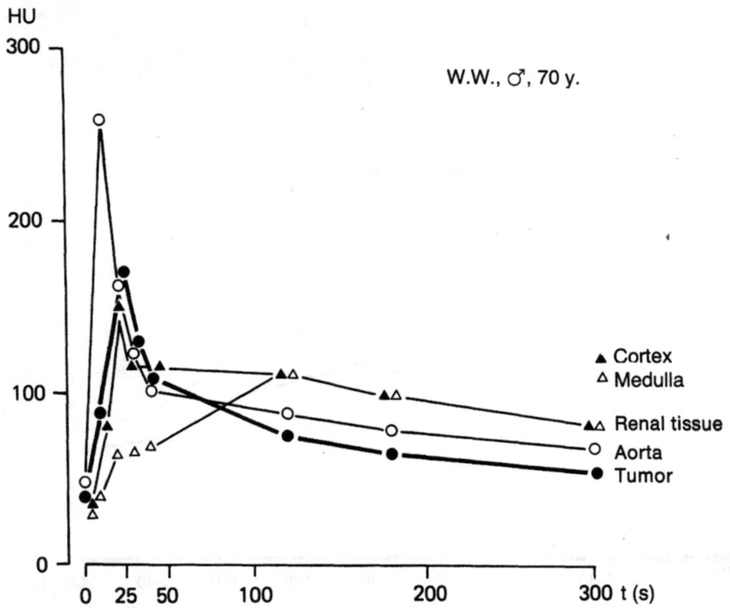

Fig. 60d

Fig. 60a–d. Renal carcinoma. **a** Isodense tumor *(arrows)* in the plain scan. **b** Demonstration of hypervascularization shortly after bolus injection followed **c** by a rapid decrease in density within the tumor, which appears hypodense in contrast to normal renal tissue. **d** Time-density diagrams

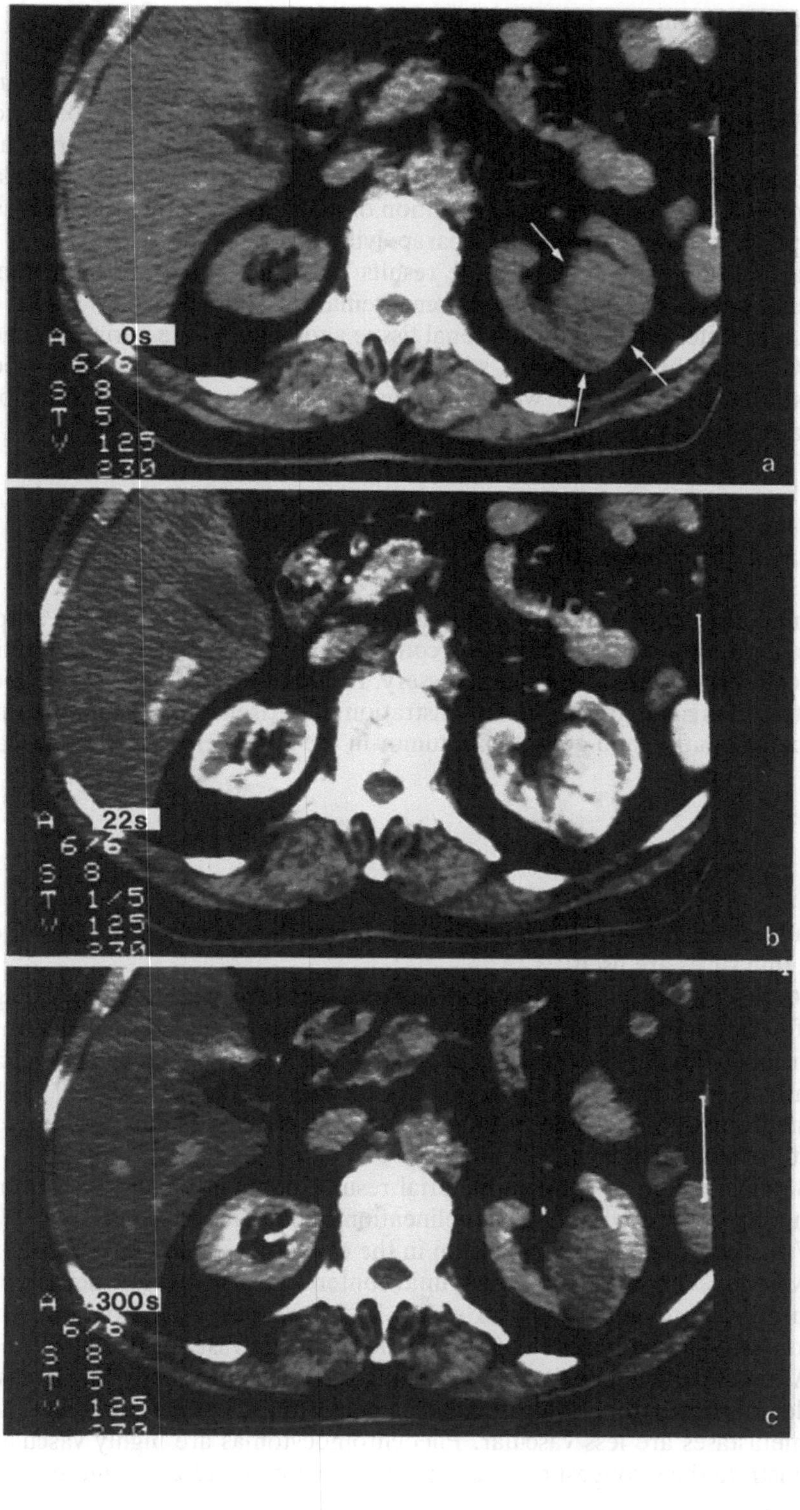
A 0s
6/6
S 8
T 5
V 125
230
a
A 22s
6/6
S 8
T 1/5
W 125
b
A 300s
6/6
S 8
T 5
W 125
c

6.8.1.4 Miscellaneous Renal Lesions

Renal cysts are usually well delineated in plain CT scans, but differential diagnosis may be difficult when density values are relatively high due to the presence of protein or cells within the cyst. Serial CT studies and time-density curves aid in differentiation between a cyst with secondary hemorrhage and a neoplasm. Dynamic CT studies allow clear definition of normal hilar structures such as the renal pelvis and vessels in cases of parapelvine cysts.

Laceration of the renal capsule results in extravasation of blood into the perirenal space, though the hematoma remains within Gerota's fascia. It is difficult to differentiate between renal tissue and blood in the perirenal space in plain CT scans, but dynamic CT studies provide better delineation of the kidney against the *hematoma* as well as a rough evaluation of renal function in comparison with the contralateral kidney.

6.8.1.5 Critical Evaluation

Dynamic CT studies permit demonstration of the vascularity of a space-occupying lesion without resort to conventional angiography, and additional diagnostic procedures may be unnecessary. In addition, CT studies are as good as or better than angiography in demonstration of perirenal extension of a tumor, lymphadenopathy, and growth of a tumor in the renal vein and the vena cava.

6.8.2 Adrenal Glands

The adrenal glands are demonstrated in plain CT scans in 95%–100% of cases when thin slices are used.

Studies with intravenous contrast material do not provide additional diagnostic information in cases of hypoplasia or hyperplasia of the adrenal glands.

Problems may arise in *delineation* of the adrenal glands against adjacent organs and structures such as the poles of the kidney, the right lobe of the liver, and major blood vessels. For example, splenic vessels may simulate enlargement of both adrenal glands.

Bolus injection of contrast material results in enhancement of surrounding organs and vessels, which aids in delineation of the adrenal glands.

Vascularity is a decisive criterion in the evaluation of *adrenal tumors*.

Adrenal adenomas have a high lipid content, resulting in low density values which may approximate those of water. In these cases differentiation between adenoma and a cyst requires bolus injection of a contrast agent.

Adrenal cortical adenomas in Cushing's disease are usually highly vascular and demonstrate strong contrast enhancement while adenomas in Conn's disease and metastases are less vascular. Pheochromocytomas are highly vascular and demonstrate the strongest contrast enhancement of all adrenal tumors.

6.8.3 Other Retroperitoneal Space-Occupying Lesions

Tumors originating in the retroperitoneal space are rare. Dynamic CT studies do not improve definition of type and degree of malignancy, but administration of a contrast medium does demonstrate the vascularity of the tumor, which aids in differential diagnosis. Hypervascular tumors include pheochromocytoma, angiosarcoma, lymphangiosarcoma, and hemangioma.

Contrast enhancement also provides important information on the extent of tumor growth as well as relations to major blood vessels. Differentiation between neoplasms and abscesses, hematomas, lymphoceles, lymphomas, and aneurysms is facilitated by the use of contrast material.

6.9 Gastrointestinal Tract

The anatomic features of the gastrointestinal tract are generally unfavorable for CT studies. Oral administration of contrast material is the most important measure for achieving adequate intraluminal contrast.

Bolus injection of a contrast agent (1 ml/kg body weight) results in an increase in density values of approximately 50 HU in the wall of the stomach and 30 HU in the intestinal wall (Fig. 61).

Dynamic CT studies do not contribute significant additional diagnostic information. Changes in density do not permit differentiation between carcinoma of the colon and conglomerate tumors secondary to inflammatory disease. Serial CT studies are not useful in differentiating between scar tissue and recurrence of a tumor after recum amputation.

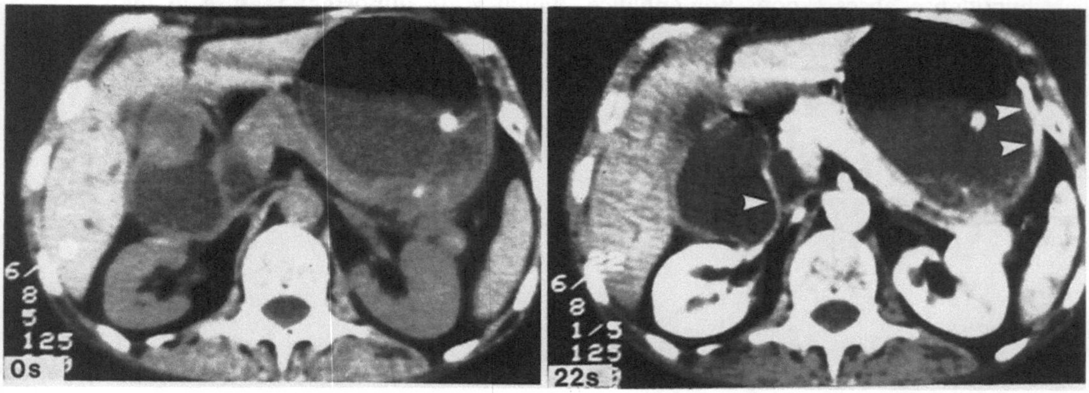

a **b**

Fig. 61. **a** Dilatation of the duodenum due to stenosis. **b** Contrast enhancement in the walls of the stomach *(arrows)* and of the duodenum *(arrow)* at 22 s

6.10 Intra-abdominal Abscess

The value of CT studies in diagnosis of abscesses is generally recognized. Presence of an abscess is likely when the following classic criteria are fulfilled:

1. A homogeneous hypodense space-occupying lesion
2. Sharply delineated walls
3. Presence of gas within the lesion
4. Displacement of adjacent organs

However, clinical findings are decisive, since these signs are unspecific. Density values within the abscess and demonstration of its walls in CT studies depend on the origin of the lesion and its stage of development. Abscesses demonstrate average density values of 10–30 HU. Fresh abscesses have density values slightly lower than normal tissue, but values decrease with liquefaction due to necrosis. Antibiotic therapy may be followed by sterilization of the abscess, resorption of the pus, and development of a cyst with high protein concentration.

CT is a sensitive technique for demonstration of very small collections of gas, which are present in 24%–42% of abscesses. Development of granulation tissue begins on the third to the fifth day after formation of the abscess, and this is significant, since contrast CT studies demonstrate significant enhancement in highly vascular granulation tissue. A hypervascular border is found in 40%–50% of all extraparenchymal abscesses (Fig. 62).

Infusion of contrast material is useful in delineation of abscesses in soft tissue, especially in cases of relatively fresh lesions with practically isodense values in the plain scan. On the other hand, conventional infusion of a contrast agent often masks the presence of a highly vascular border in the abscess. This is the special province of dynamic CT studies, which demonstrate selective arterial contrast enhancement in the membrane of the abscess. Problems in differential diagnosis arise in discrimination between necrotic metastases and abscesses with wide irregular membranes. Time-density curves demonstrate that the initially hypodense abscess does not enhance, which is an important feature in discriminating between an abscess and a solid tumor.

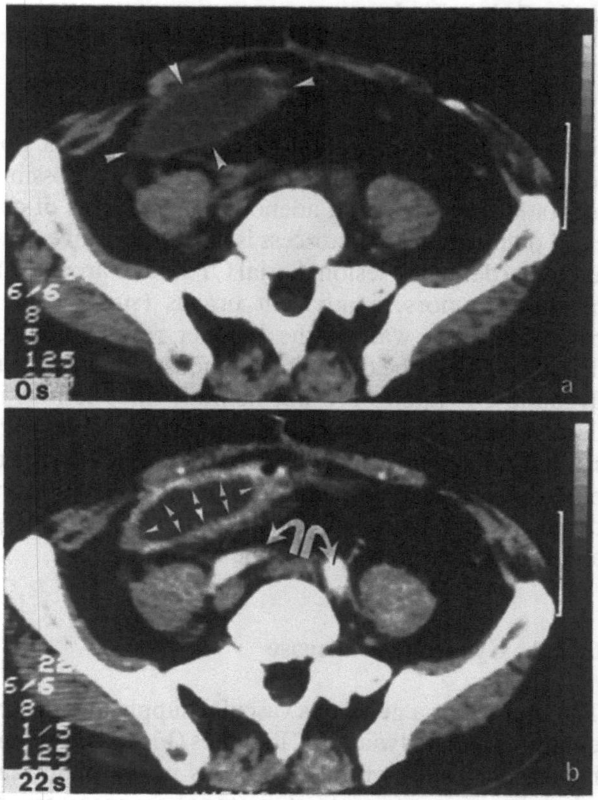

Fig. 62. **a** Abscess in the lower abdomen on the right after resection of a non-Hodgkin lymphoma (H. K., male, 57 years). An 8×4 cm hypodense space-occupying lesion is demonstrated below the abdominal wall. **b** A hyperdense border of contrast enhancement representing the capsule of the abscess appears after administration of a contrast agent. Both iliac arteries are demonstrated *(arrows)*

6.11 Pelvic Lesions

6.11.1 Neoplasms of the Prostate and the Bladder

Intravenous administration of contrast material does not improve diagnostic results in disease of the prostate. It is not possible to differentiate between prostatic carcinoma and adenoma on the basis of contrast enhancement. However, delineation of an abscess is improved, since contrast enhancement is strong at the border of the lesion. Serial CT studies are not diagnostic in neoplasms of the bladder. Tumors in adjacent organs (such as the prostate and the uterus) penetrating the wall of the bladder result in major problems in differential diagnosis. It may be difficult to demonstrate the primary tumor in some cases, and dynamic CT studies are not helpful, since lesions in the pelvic region do not demonstrate significant changes in density values suggestive of a specific diagnosis. It is not possible to diagnose pelvic tumors in the retroperitoneal space on the basis of contrast enhancement if their relations to normal organs are not demonstrated. However, CT studies do aid in defining the extent of tumor growth and the vascular relations of the lesion.

6.11.2 Gynecologic Disease

The uterus has a generous vascular supply and demonstrates significant contrast enhancement in dynamic CT studies (Fig. 63). Endometrial carcinomas appear as hypodense zones within the uterus in the plain scan in advanced disease, but administration of contrast material is necessary for demonstration of early endometrial carcinoma. These lesions appear as low-density zones within the hyperdense wall of the uterus, which allows definition of the extent of myometrial infiltration. Time-density curves aid in differentiation of endometrial carcinoma from intracavitary blood or pus in the uterus, since the latter do not enhance, while endometrial carcinoma usually demonstrates an increase of 10 HU after administration of contrast material.

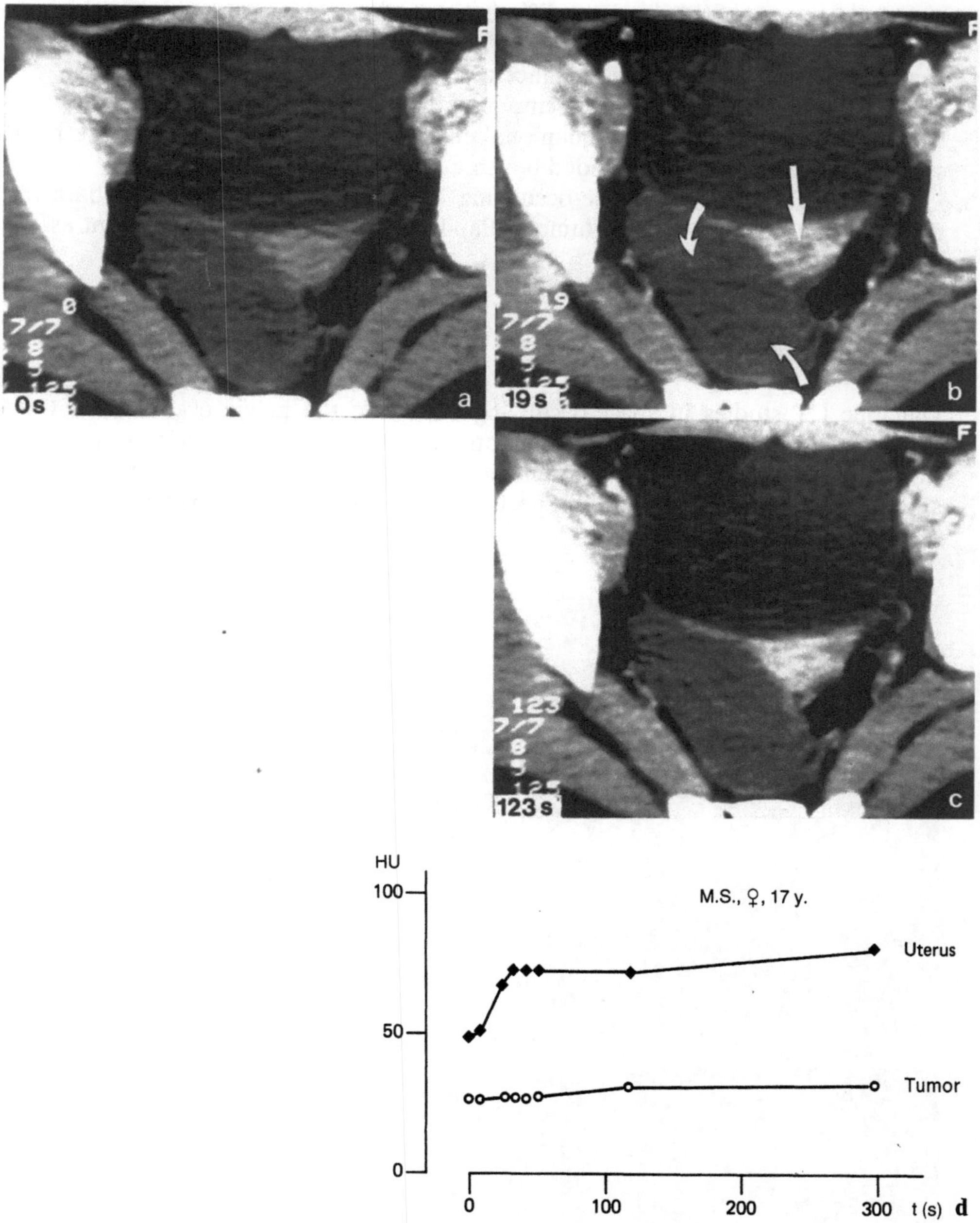

Fig. 63 a–d. Neurofibroma in the pelvis. 8×4×7 cm oval, sharply delineated tumor in the right pelvis. Homogeneous density values (25 HU) with gradual slight increase in enhancement at 1 min *(curved arrow)*. The uterus *(arrow)* demonstrates early and persistent contrast enhancement

Myomas are usually easily differentiated from space-occupying pelvic lesions, even when the former fail to demonstrate calcification, since they generally show strong contrast enhancement with nodular structures (Fig. 64).

Demonstration of cervical carcinoma is not improved in contrast studies, because diffuse infiltration by squamous cell carcinoma escapes detection in CT scans if the lesion has not extended beyond the uterus.

Solid highly vascular space-occupying lesions are demonstrated in both malignant and benign ovarian tumors. Papillary cystadenomas may present as highly vascular tumors.

6.11.3 Critical Evaluation

Dynamic CT studies in space-occupying lesions of the pelvic organs do not provide significant additional information, except in gynecologic disease. Infusion of contrast material results in enhancement within the major pelvic vessels and the ureters, and this method is preferred in CT studies of the pelvic region.

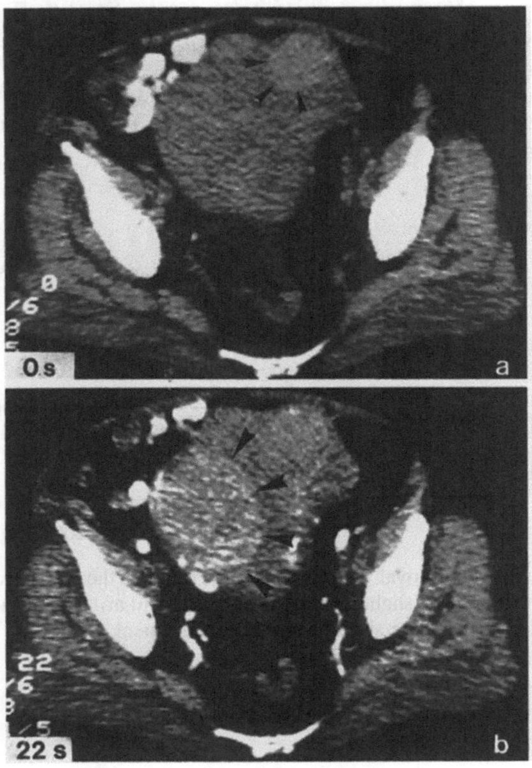

Fig. 64a, b. Uterine myoma. **a** Demonstration of a hyperdense myoma *(arrows)* at the ventral border of the enlarged uterus in the plain CT scan. **b** Administration of a contrast agent reveals a second large intramural myoma *(arrows)*

6.12 Soft Tissue Lesions

CT studies aid in defining the location and extent of soft tissue lesions, and specific diagnoses may be possible in lipomas, for example. Isodense tumors present greater problems. Bolus injection of contrast material allows demonstration of the extent and location of tumor growth in muscles and beyond, and the tumor's relations to major vessels are revealed.

Demonstration of the vascularity of a structure provides information useful in the differential dagnosis of space-occupying soft tissue lesions. For example, strong enhancement after bolus injection suggests a diagnosis of hemangioma or angiosarcoma.

Malignant lesions with rapid growth, necrosis, edema, and hemorrhage may show strong enhancement at their borders. However, differentiation between these lesions and hematomas or abscesses on the basis of their appearance in plain scans or after contrast enhancement may prove impossible. Well delineated malignant tumors with large central zones of necrosis may simulate abscesses in CT studies.

6.13 Cranial Computed Tomography

The earliest cranial CT studies revealed that meningiomas demonstrate contrast enhancement approximately 2 h after carotid angiography, and use of contrast material has become indispensable in CT studies. The brain is unique in that contrast material does not pass from the intravascular to the interstitial space under normal conditions. A number of factors collectively termed the blood-brain barrier are responsible for this phenomenon:

1. A barrier for macromolecules located in the capillaries and the endothelium of the choroid plexus
2. Cell membranes
3. Selective ion regulation
4. Transport mechanisms in capillary endothelium
5. Selective resorption of ions and organic acids by the choroid plexus

In principle, iodine might pass from the vascular space to the interstitial space in normal brain tissue as a result of the hyperosmolarity of the contrast material.

Administration of high doses of contrast material is followed by passage into the interstitial space as a result of a disorder of autoregulation and changes in viscosity and hematocrit. Brain disease causes disorders in the blood-brain barrier, with passage of contrast material to the extravascular space.

6.13.1 Normal Regional Circulation

Transit of contrast material typically involves four phases:

1. A slow wash-in phase with a 20%–30% increase in density at 5–10 s
2. A rapid wash-in phase with a 65%–70% increase in density values at 10–19 s
3. A rapid wash-out phase with a 60%–70% decline in density at 19–25 s
4. A slow wash-out phase with a decrease in density of 30%–40% after 25 s

The same contrast material is used for CT studies of the brain and the abdomen.

6.13.2 Vascular Studies

Dynamic CT studies with small doses of contrast material result in better demonstration of brain vessels and vascular malformations (Fig. 65) than does continuous infusion of contrast material. Conventional angiography is necessary for demonstration of small vessels, but CT provides outstanding visualization of the internal carotid artery, the arteries at the base of the skull, the basilar artery, the middle cerebral artery, and the anterior cerebral artery with their main branches. The large veins and sinuses are also clearly defined.

Fig. 65. **a** Contrast enhancement in a patient with a vascular anomaly in the left parieto-occipital ▶ region. The center of the arteriovenous malformation is *region 4,* while *region 5* designates adjacent brain tissue. Perfusion analysis in the gray matter *(region 7)* and white matter *(region 6)* was performed in contralateral brain tissue. There is a 1:3 ratio in brain perfusion between white and gray matter in the normal right hemisphere, corresponding to known physiologic values for cerebral circulation. There is a significant increase in density within the angioma in the left hemisphere at 15 s; the values are considerably higher than in normal brain tissue. **b** Demonstration of the relations within the vascular anomaly and in adjacent brain tissue. Reduced perfusion in adjacent tissue is attributed to a steal effect, while there is pronounced hyperperfusion in the center of the vascular abnormality. At 5 min density values within the angioma remain slightly higher than normal. This suggests the presence of contrast material which has passed from the intravascular space to the interstitial space

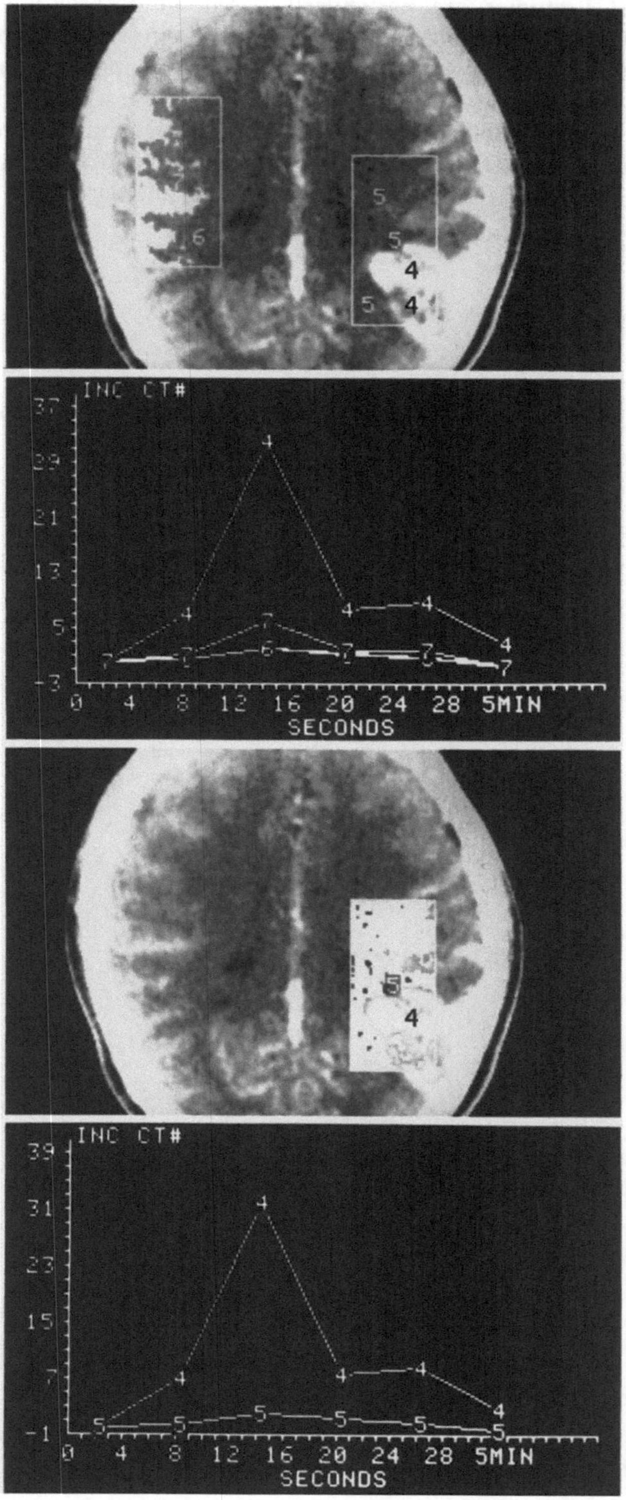

6
5
5
4
5
4
INC CT#
37
29
21
13
5
-3
0 4 8 12 16 20 24 28 5MIN
SECONDS
5
4
INC CT#
39
31
23
15
7
-1
0 4 8 12 16 20 24 28 5MIN
SECONDS

a

b

Dynamic CT studies are particularly useful in differentiation between aneurysm and tumor. For example, aneurysms in the circle of Willis may simulate pituitary adenomas. Aneurysms and angiomas (Fig. 66) appear at the same time and with the same density as the intracranial arteries, while highly vascular tumors such as meningiomas are associated with high but delayed peaks of contrast enhancement. Differentiation between aneurysm and angioma is not possible with dynamic CT studies, and conventional angiography is necessary to this purpose.

Fig. 66a–c. Angiomatosis of the basilar artery. In the arterial phase there is rapid and extensive filling ▶ of coiled vessels

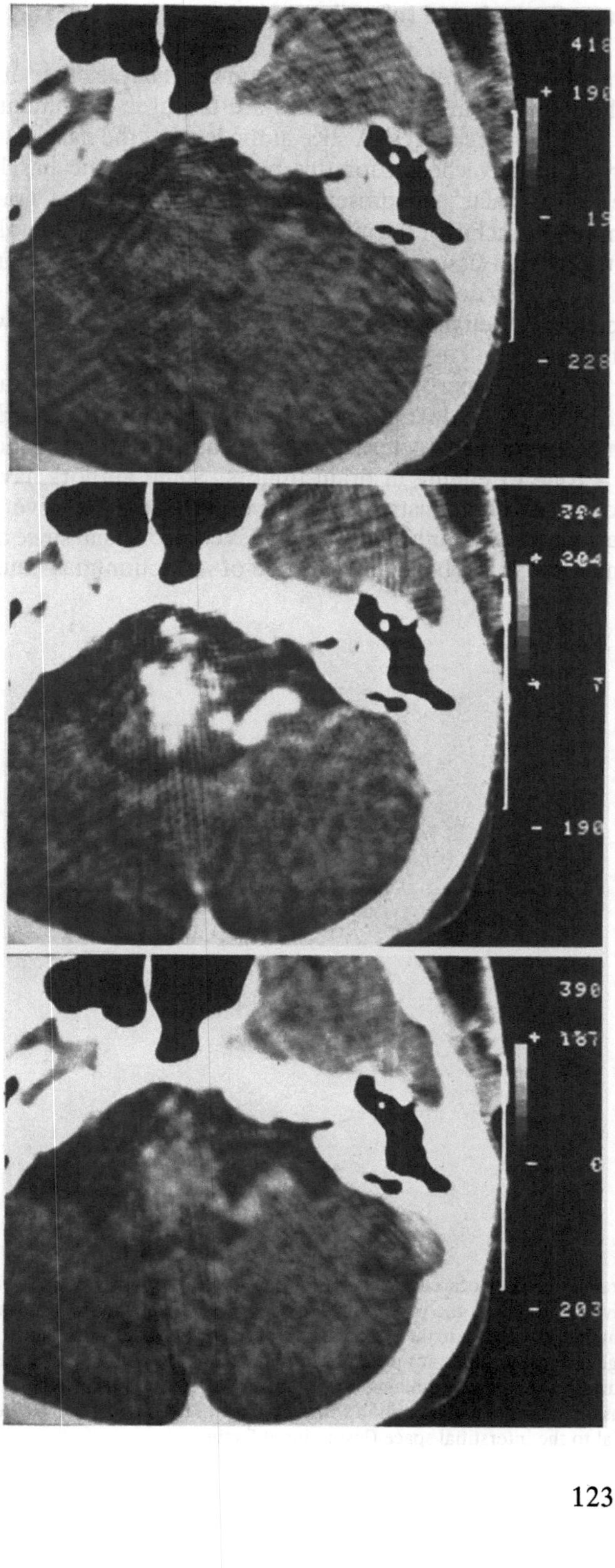

a
b
c

6.13.3 Vascular Stenosis and Infarction

Dynamic CT studies permit evaluation of the functional relevance of extracranial stenoses of the internal carotid artery and are useful in documenting vascular patency after surgical procedures. A slice at the level of the basal ganglia and the sylvian fissure is usually chosen for this purpose, since the basal ganglia are relatively free of artifacts and present well defined zones of gray and white matter. The major branches of the middle cerebral artery are generally parallel to the plane of the sylvian fissure. Calculation of mean transit time and corrected mean transit time can demonstrate perfusion disorders as well as adequate collateral circulation. Reliable results are possible only in patients with an intact blood-brain barrier.

Hypoperfusion or hyperperfusion may be demonstrated in brain infarction (Fig. 67) with or without disruption of the blood-brain barrier. Extravascular accumulation of iodine is characteristic of brain infarction, which allows differentiation from a zone of edema in brain tumors. Some authors have assigned a favorable prognosis to demonstration of hyperperfusion. However, administration of contrast material after brain infarction is controversial since accumulation of contrast material at the borders of a zone of infarction may cause additional damage.

Fig. 67 a, b. Brain infarction located in the internal capsule and the anterior basal ganglia on the left ▶ *(arrow)*. **a** Individual stages of the perfusion study with visible enhancement in the major vessels. **b** Analysis of time-density curves in the region of infarction *(region 0)* and in adjacent tissue *(1)* reveals significantly higher density values at the center of the zone of infarction than in the periphery. The time-density curve at the center remains above normal at 5 min. This suggests the presence of increased perfusion in the zone of infarction with a disorder of the blood-brain barrier and passage of contrast material to the interstitial space (last point at 5 min)

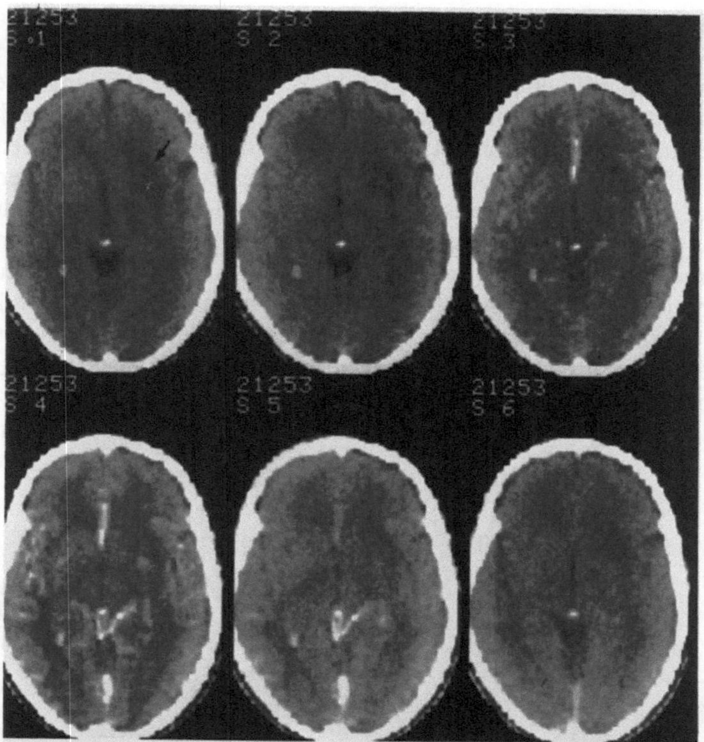
21253
S 1
21253
S 2
21253
S 3
21253
S 4
21253
S 5
21253
S 6

a

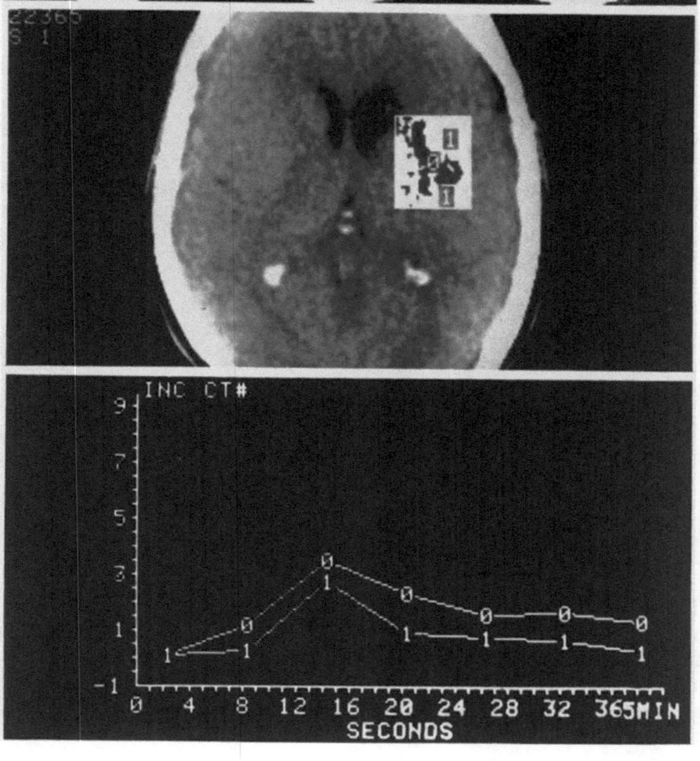
22365
S 1
INC CT#
9
7
5
3
1
-1
0 4 8 12 16 20 24 28 32 36 5MIN
SECONDS

b

6.13.4 Tumors and Brain Edema

The density values in edema and brain infarction may be similar in the plain CT scan. Hypoperfusion and slight extravasation of contrast material are characteristic of edema. Differentiation between edema and infarction is most readily made in the wash-out phase, since significant passage of contrast material to the interstitial space is characteristic of brain infarction. Hyperperfusion in solid tumors is secondary to vasodilation and increased vascularity. Time-density curves may reveal both a vascular component and an extravascular effect secondary to disruption of the blood-brain barrier (Fig. 68). Studies of the kinetics of contrast material in cerebral tumors have shown that a number of lesions take up contrast material to various degrees, but the wide range in density values makes diagnosis of specific tumors rather difficult (Lange et al. 1979). These results were obtained with conventional CT studies made several minutes

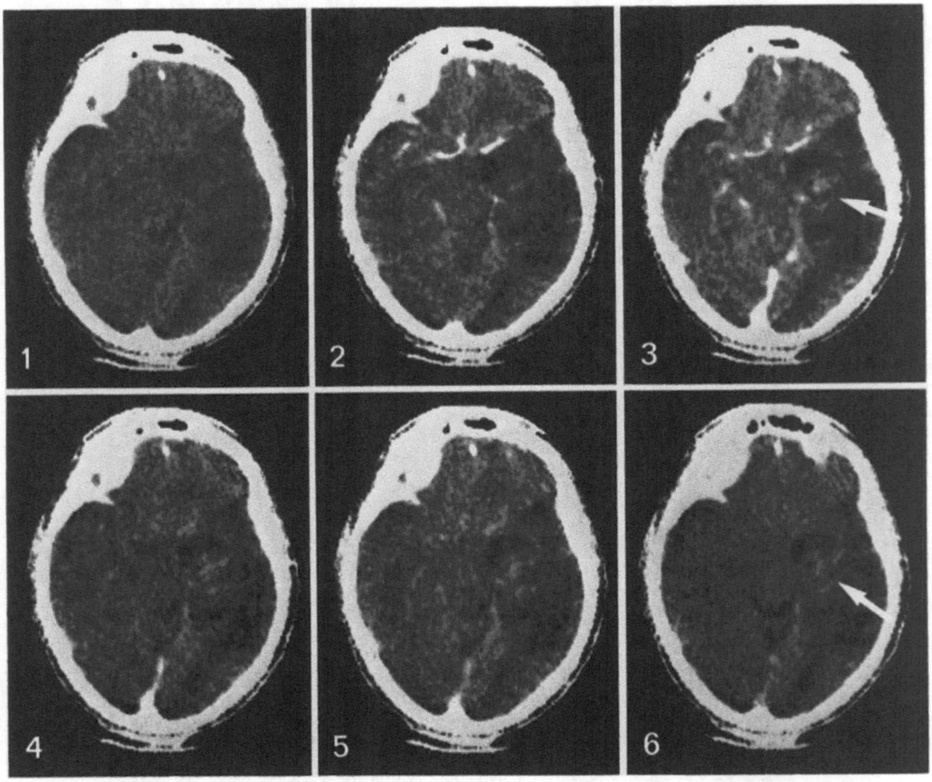

Fig. 68. Extensive glioblastoma in the right temporoparietal region. **1** plain scan; **2** significant increase in density values in the major vessels of the circle of Willis; **3** highly vascular zone at the center of the tumor *(arrow)* with a **4, 5** subsequent decrease in density and **6** passage of contrast medium to the interstitial space *(arrow)* due to a disorder of the blood-brain barrier at 5 min. This case demonstrates the relationship between highly vascular tumors and adjacent brain tissue as well as the relation of major vessels to the tumor itself

after intravenous administration of contrast material. Dynamic CT studies in the first minute after bolus injection demonstrate the vascularity of a tumor, but enhancement in most cerebral tumors is related to passage of contrast material to the interstitial space of the tumor. As a result, conventional CT studies with infusion of contrast material are prefered to dynamic CT studies in the diagnosis of intracranial lesions. Cysts usually show hypoperfusion as a result of connective tissue elements, small blood vessels, and slight extravasation of contrast material.

6.13.5 Blood Volume and Circulation

Contrast CT studies allow determinations of regional blood volume on the basis of differences in attenuation values before and after administration of contrast material, with external measurements of the concentration of the contrast agent in the blood and hematocrit determinations. Cerebral circulation can also be calculated from the corrected transit time of the first passage of contrast material if the temporal resolution of the CT system is less than 1 s. However, these studies are difficult and are comparable to those obtained with other methods only when the blood-brain barrier is intact.

6.13.6 Critical Evaluation

Dynamic cranial CT studies have not attained the same importance as in other regions of the body, since other methods such as scintigraphy offer better temporal resolution and are more appropriate for studies of the brain. Conventional CT studies using intravenous infusion of approximately 300 mg iodine/kg body weight are usually effective in demonstration and differentiation of pathologic processes. Contrast studies with doses as high as 80 g iodine may be made for resolution of specific problems, such as exclusion of multiple small brain metastases when neurosurgical therapy is contemplated.

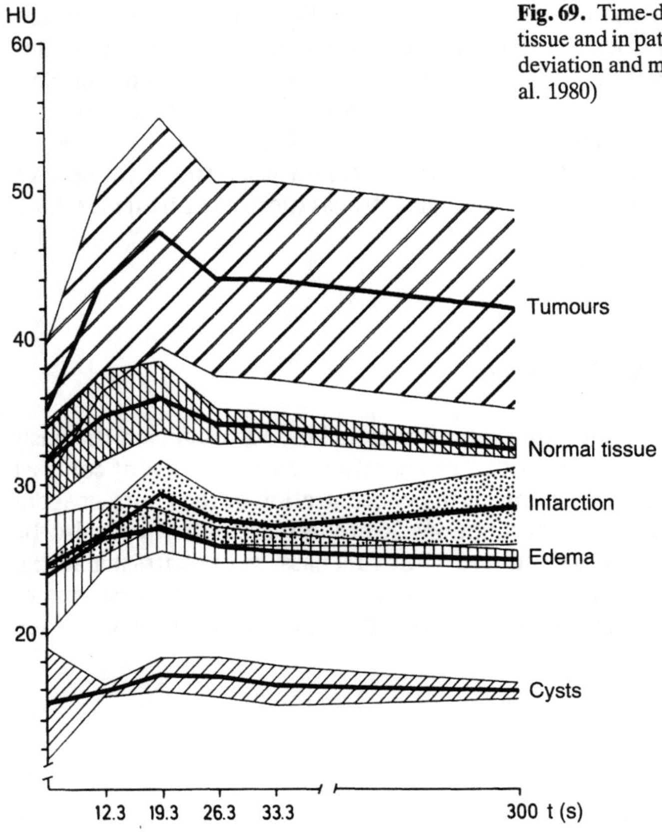

Fig. 69. Time-density curves in normal brain tissue and in pathologic conditions. Standard deviation and mean values. (After Traupe et al. 1980)

Traupe et al. (1980) summarized the present role of dynamic cranial CT studies as follows (Fig. 69):

1. Differentiation between hyperperfusion and extravasation on the basis of time-density relationships in the first 5 min.
2. Demonstration of hypoperfusion and slight extravasation in edema and cystic lesions, which permits differentiation from brain infarction.
3. Demonstration of hypoperfusion or hyperperfusion with or without disruption of the blood-brain barrier in brain infarction. Hyperperfusion is considered a prognostically favorable sign.
4. Differentiation between intravascular and extravascular contrast enhancement.
5. Optimum demonstration of brain vessels and small cerebral lesions with low iodine concentrations.
6. Determinations of blood volume and brain perfusion, though these studies are unreliable when disruption of the blood-brain barrier is present.
7. Evaluation of the functional significance of extracranial stenosis of the carotid and vertebral areries; evaluation of vascular patency following surgical procedures.

8. Differentiation between aneurysm and tumors with strong contrast enhancement on the basis of time-density relationships.

6.14 Orbits

The differences in attenuation values between fat in the orbital space and adjacent intraorbital structures are significantly greater than those encountered in most other body regions. As a result, the normal orbit is an ideal location for demonstration of a space-occupying lesion with CT studies. Intravenous administration of contrast material is followed by an increase in the density gradient between orbital fat and muscles, blood vessels, and nerves located in the orbit, but this increase in density is slight when compared with the differences evident in the plain scan. For this reason there are few indications for contrast studies of the orbit.

6.14.1 Normal Findings with Contrast Media

There is a significant increase in contrast enhancement in the wall of the eyeball (15 ± 4 HU) and the optic nerve (11 ± 3 HU) after intravenous administration of 150 ml of a triiodinated 60% contrast agent over a period of 3–4 min. The external ocular muscles also show contrast enhancement averaging 41 HU (Watanabe et al. 1982), which differs significantly from normal skeletal muscle in other regions of the body. For example, the temporal muscle exhibits maximum contrast enhancement of 20 HU. This is explained by characteristic differences in the histologic structures and metabolism of the ocular muscles.

The small volume of the orbital structures and ocular motion may result in false density measurements in dynamic CT studies.

Bolus injection of 50 ml of contrast material is followed by an increase in density values within the wall of the eyeball averaging 8 HU.

6.14.2 Pathologic Findings

Malignant melanomas arising in the choroid present as hyperdense tumors with density values averaging 64.6 HU in the plain scan. Bolus injection of contrast material results in enhancement ranging from 72 to 115 HU, an average increase in density values of 17.2 HU (Heller et al. 1982) (Fig. 70).

Choroidal metastases and inflammatory pseudotumors are not associated with the same degree of contrast enhancement.

Optic nerve gliomas demonstrate less enhancement than do meningiomas of the optic nerve sheath.

Suspicion of a carotid–cavernous sinus fistula is an indication for contrast studies, since the latter are often necessary for demonstration of the lesion.

6.14.3 Critical Evaluation

Contrast material is usually unnecessary in studies of orbital structures when a CT system with high resolution and thin slices (5 mm) is used, since contrast studies usually provide little additional information.

Suspicion of malignant melanoma in the choroid is an indication for contrast studies when ophthalmoscopic examination is inadequate due to hemorrhage in the vitreous humor.

6.15 Face and Neck

The introduction of whole body CT scanning provided a major advance in the diagnosis of lesions in the facial skull. CT allows excellent demonstration of the complex anatomic relations in this region. A wide range of structures is visualized, including the paranasal sinuses, which contain air, areas such as the retromaxillary and parapharyngeal spaces composed of soft tissues, and bone structures such as the facial skull, the base of the skull, the orbits, and the cranium. Even small pathologic processes are demonstrated in horizontal and frontal CT slices, and characteristic extension of tumors arising in the nasal cavity, the paranasal sinuses, and the retromaxillary space into bone and soft tissue structures with penetration of the orbits, the base of the skull, and the intracranial cavity is visible. CT provides the means for exact staging and optimal planning of therapeutic strategies.

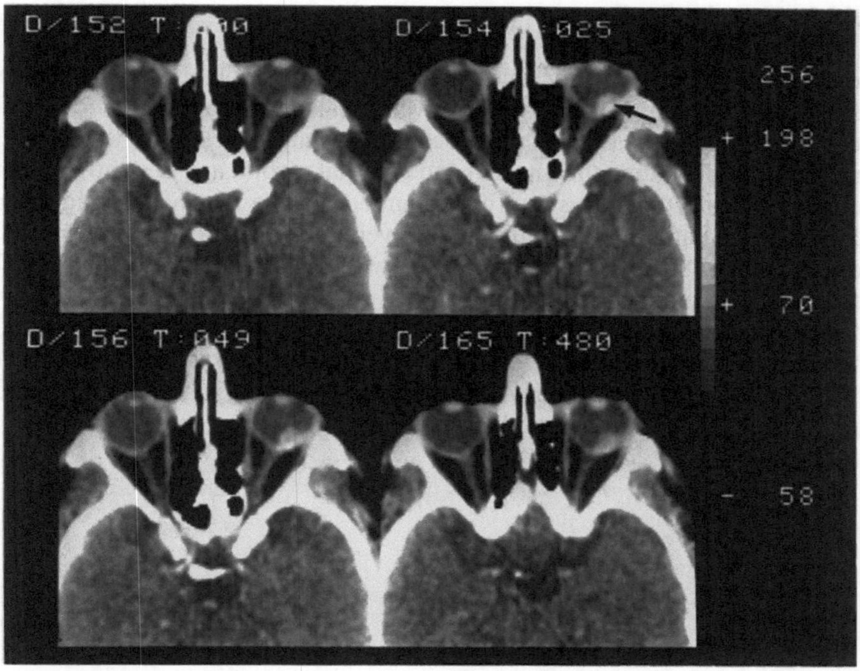

Fig. 70. Choroidal melanoma near the right macula. Serial CT studies at 0, 25, 49, and 480 s. Maximum contrast enhancement at 25 s *(arrow)*. (Heller et al. 1982)

6.15.1 Vascular Studies

Few regions in the body offer such a complex juxtaposition of arterial and venous vessels as does the facial skull. Conventional angiography is necessary for demonstration and analysis of small vessels. The major vessels of the facial skull and the neck, including the internal and external carotid arteries and the jugular veins, are clearly demonstrated by dynamic CT. The internal carotid artery is located ventral and medial to the jugular vein in the craniovertebral space, and compression of the internal carotid artery with occlusion of the jugular vein by a retromaxillary tumor is evident in contrast studies (Fig. 71). The maxillary and facial arteries, which are branches of the external carotid artery, and corresponding veins in this region are also visible. Infusion of contrast material and bolus injection are capable of demonstrating hypervascularization in the mucous membranes of the mouth and pharynx.

Fig. 71 a–d. Undifferentiated carcinoma in the retromaxillary and parapharyngeal spaces on the left ▶ (J.D., male, 55 years). **a** Horizontal slice through the nasopharynx, maxillary sinuses, the nasal cavity, and the retromaxillary space. **b** Demonstration of the internal carotid artery (↙) and the internal jugular vein (↖) in their typical locations. The left internal jugular vein is not demonstrated since it has been compressed by the tumor, while the left internal carotid artery is displaced laterally to a position anterior to the styloid process (↘). **c** Time-density diagrams. **d** Follow-up study at 4 weeks following irradiation with 5000 rad. There is a significant increase in density values in muscle as compared with CT studies before radiation therapy. There is little change in density values within the tumor in the second phase, and there is no density gradient between the intravascular and interstitial spaces

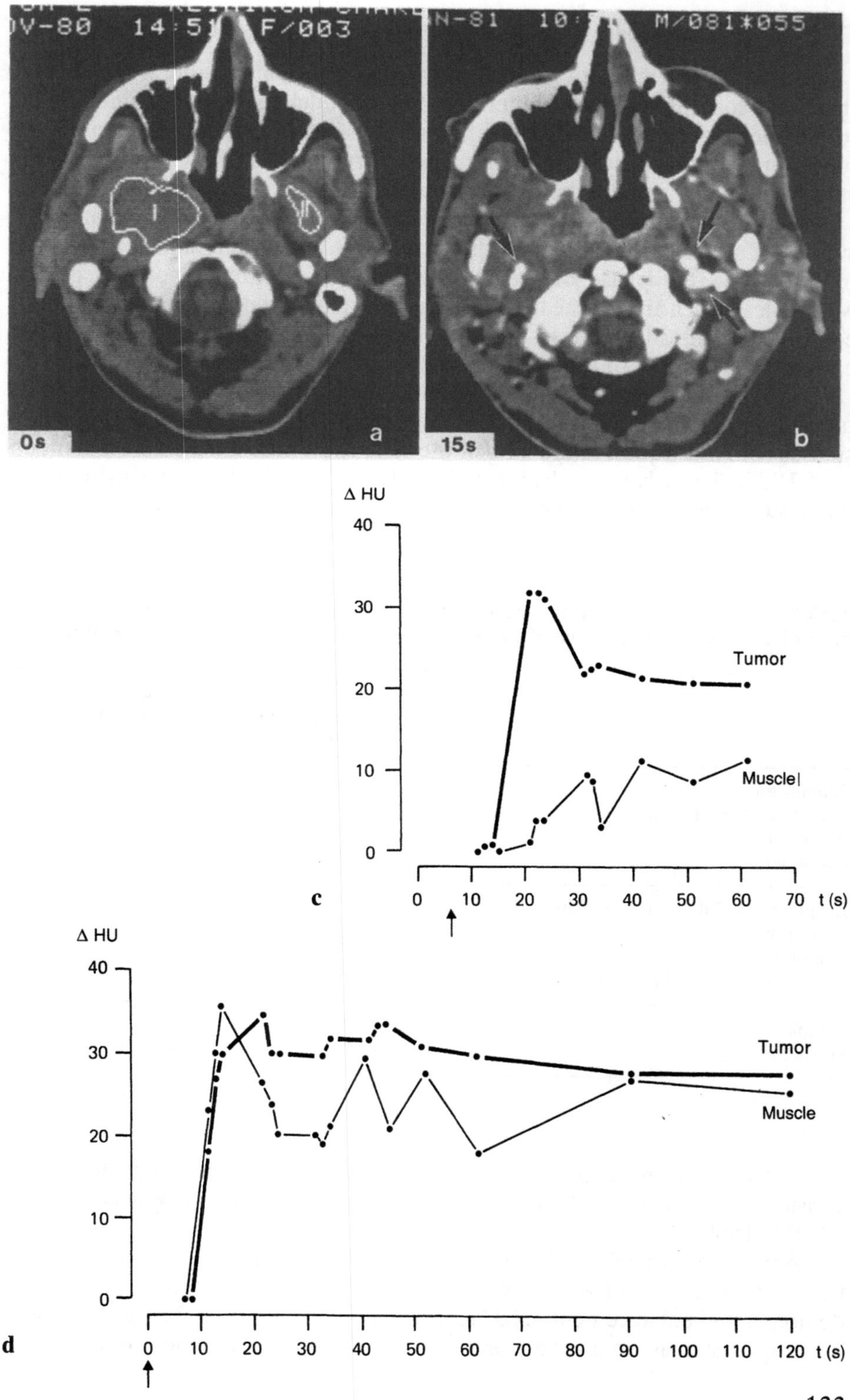

0V-80 14:51 F/003
N-81 10:5 M/081*055
0s
a
15s
b
Δ HU
40
30
20
10
0
Tumor
Muscle I
0 10 20 30 40 50 60 70 t (s)
c
Δ HU
40
30
20
10
0
Tumor
Muscle
0 10 20 30 40 50 60 70 80 90 100 110 120 t (s)
d

6.15.2 Tumors

Tumors in the soft tissues of the retromaxillary space are visible when normal structures containing fat are obliterated, but exact delineation of a tumor within soft tissues often requires administration of contrast material. In some cases tumors in the parapharyngeal and retromaxillary spaces are revealed by demonstration of highly vascular borders after administration of contrast material.

Table 3 illustrates maximum contrast enhancement achieved in dynamic CT studies of a number of tumors in the facial skull. Maximum enhancement was found during the phase of greatest perfusion in all tumors of this group. Mucoceles, which arise in the frontal sinuses and may extend through the ethmoid cells into the maxillary sinuses, do not enhance. Lymphoblastoma shows slight enhancement similar to that found in the muscles of the facial skull.

Juvenile fibromas of the nasal cavity and pharynx as well as differentiated and undifferentiated carcinomas arising in the retromaxillary space and the maxillary sinuses with infiltration of the base of the skull show maximum enhancement up to 30 HU in the early phase. This is followed by a rapid decrease in density values and a subsequent gradual decrease in attenuation up to 180 s (Table 3).

Table 3. Changes in contrast enhancement (Δ HU) following intravenous administration of contrast material in space-occupying lesions of the facial skull (1 ml/kg body weight, flow rate 8 ml/s)

	Increase in density in the early phase (10–30 s) Δ HU	Decrease in density (40–60 s) Δ HU
Glomus tumor	> 100	> 50
Metastatic thyroid carcinoma	> 50	> 30
Angiofibroma	30–50	> 15
Carcinomas	30–50	> 15
Lymphoepithelial carcinoma (Schmincke's tumor) Carcinoma Cylindroma Juvenile fibroma of the pharynx	20–30	> 10
Lymphoblastoma	< 10	< 5
Mucocele	< 5	—

Carcinomas and angiofibromas are characterized by a rapid increase in density averaging 30–50 HU in the arterial phase, followed by a rapid decrease of 30 HU (Table 3).

A metastasis of a thyroid carcinoma which did not retain iodine was located in the soft tissues of the oropharynx and the upper cervical region on the left side and demonstrated enhancement of 80 HU in the first 25 s (Fig. 72). This was followed by a rapid decrease in attenuation of 25–30 HU in the subsequent few seconds,

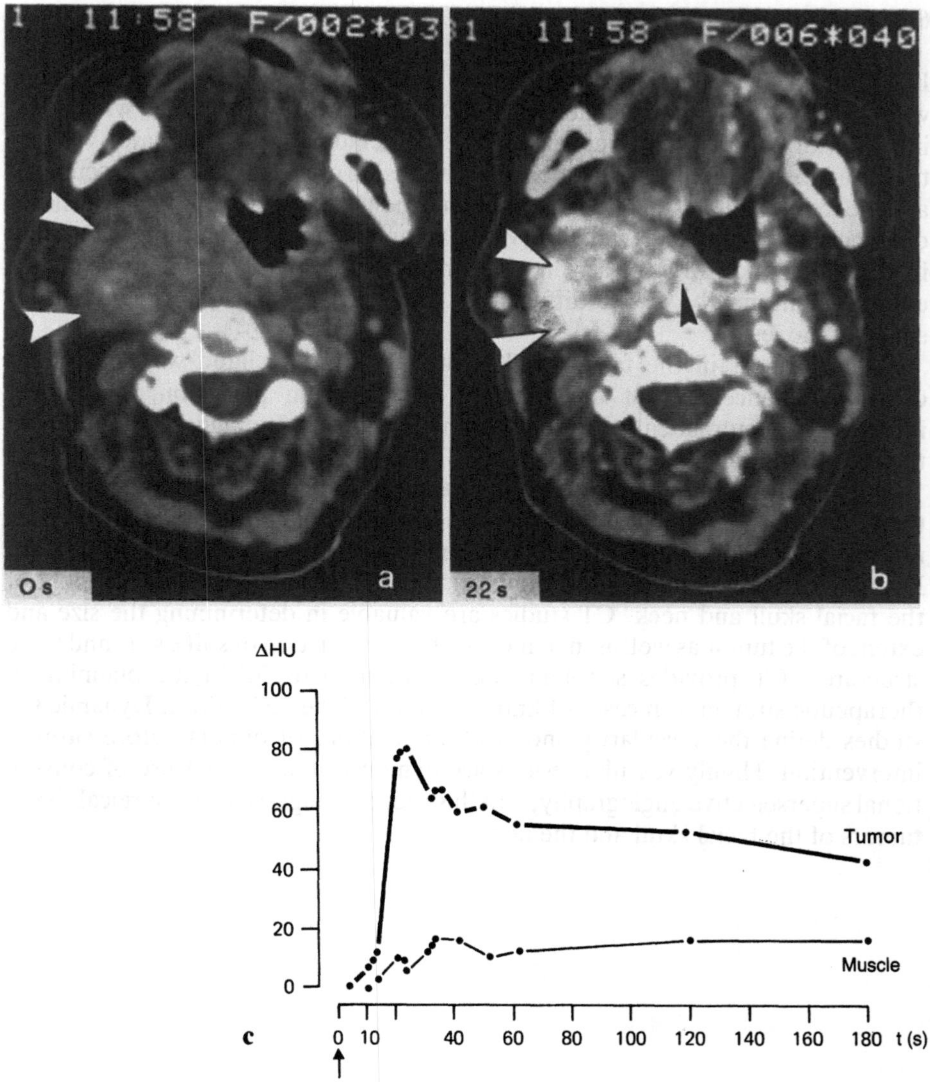

Fig. 72 a–c. Metastasis of a papillary and follicular thyroid carcinoma located in the oropharynx on the left. Serial CT studies **a** before contrast administration and **b** at 22 s. Significant enhancement within the tumor, which has spread around the pharynx from the left and dorsal *(arrows)*. **c** Time-density diagrams

with a further gradual decrease in density over the following 3 min, which resulted in a contrast gradient of 40 HU. Glomus tumors were associated with extreme increases in density values averaging more than 100 HU shortly after enhancement of the carotid artery, followed by decreases in attenuation which were almost as rapid as those in the major vessels during the first 60 s (Table 3).

6.15.3 Critical Evaluation

Localization of a space-occupying lesion in the facial skull is usually possible without resort to contrast material in CT scans. Serial CT studies with bolus injection of contrast material are capable of demonstrating the major vessels, their relations to tumors, displacement or occlusion of vessels, and the vascularity and degree of interstitial contrast enhancement within a tumor. This allows differentiation of avascular, slightly vascular, and highly vascular tumors. A delay in the elimination of contrast material from a tumor after maximum contrast enhancement may be due to diffusion of the contrast agent into the interstitial space of the lesion.

Most tumors in the facial skull, however, are associated with maximum contrast enhancement at the moment of maximum perfusion. Therefore, intravascular contrast enhancement is of major interest in diagnosis of tumors in the facial skull.

Generally speaking, glomus tumors, angiofibromas, and most metastases in the facial skull are highly vascular tumors. Analysis of time-density relations does not provide reliable diagnostic information in most other tumors of this region. Histologic studies of material obtained at biopsy are usually available in lesions of the facial skull and neck. CT studies are valuable in determining the size and extent of the tumor as well as in demonstrating destruction of soft tissue and bone structures. CT provides supplemental information useful in the planning of therapeutic strategies in cases of known tumors of the facial skull. Dynamic CT studies define the vascularity and vascular relations of tumors before surgical intervention. Highly vascular lesions are demonstrated without use of conventional superselective angiography, and this reduces diagnostic and surgical risk in tumors of the facial skull and the neck.

7 Summary

Contrast enhancement reaches its maximum in parenchymal organs during the first circulatory cycle, and peak enhancement is a function of perfusion within the organ in question. Density values in parenchymal organs in the early phase are related primarily to contrast enhancement within the blood vessels.

Systematic studies by a number of groups have shown that there are no major differences between ionic and nonionic contrast agents during the first passage through a given organ and in later phases of distribution. Differences in physicochemical characteristics of conventional contrast agents are so slight that there is no significant difference in contrast enhancement or time-density relations with a given dose of contrast material, although there are differences in osmotic pressure, viscosity, and molecular weight among the products. Contrast agents with low osmotic pressure are not associated with significant differences in time-density curves for contrast studies in blood vessels and parenchymatous organs, even though practically isotonic contrast agents cause less significant decreases in hematocrit than do contrast agents with higher osmotic pressure.

Contrast is increased by administration of larger doses of contrast material, and the relationship between maximum contrast enhancement and dose is nearly linear. The increase in dose may be obtained by increasing the volume or the concentration of the contrast agent. These relations obtain in blood vessels and in parenchymatous organs. The duration of maximum enhancement is prolonged with larger volumes of contrast material.

Increasing the flow rate results in an earlier and higher peak of contrast enhancement in the aorta, but increases above 8 ml/s do not result in significant increases in maximum enhancement. However, the increase in enhancement achieved with higher flow rates is less than that obtained by administration of a larger dose of contrast material. Higher flow rates do not result in significant increases in contrast enhancement in parenchymatous organs.

Our studies have shown that higher heart rates are associated with earlier peaks of contrast enhancement in the aorta. As a result, heart rate, total volume of contrast material, and flow rate must be considered in estimations of expected peak times. Even when these known relations are taken into account, intraindividual variability may result in deviations from expected peak time. Maximum contrast enhancement in the aorta may also vary from individual to individual. Increasing the contrast gradient between a circumscribed lesion and adjacent normal tissue in parenchymatous organs such as the liver and pancreas results in better delineation of the lesion.

The vascularity of circumscribed lesions may be defined without resort to conventional angiography, and the information obtained may be useful in differential diagnosis. For example, the pattern of enhancement in cavernous hemangioma of the liver is so characteristic that additional studies are unnecessary.

Time-density measurements allow definition of perfusion in organs and tissues. A reduction in contrast enhancement may be interpreted as a sign of a functional disorder.

With the introduction of modern fast systems, dynamic CT studies will play a major role in the diagnosis of space-occupying lesions and will become the noninvasive procedure of choice employed before other invasive diagnostic techniques.

The disadvantage of the technique lies in the fact that dynamic CT studies are limited to a single preselected slice, with the result that contrast enhancement in the rest of a lesion escapes examination.

Rapid CT studies in several slices offer an attractive alternative in order to demonstrate contrast enhancement in blood vessels and soft tissue in several planes, but exact time-density curves are not available with this procedure.

References

Albert SA (1971) Blood volume and extracellular fluid volume. Thomas, Springfield

Ansell G (1970) Adverse reactions to contrast agents. Invest Radiol 5:374–384

Araki T, Itai Y, Furui S, Tasaka A (1980) Dynamic CT densitometry of hepatic tumors. AJR 135:1037–1043

Ariyama J, Shirakabe H, Shimaguchi S, Autenrieht J (1980) Kritischer Vergleich der Untersuchungsmethoden bei der Frage nach einem Pankreaskarzinom. RöFo 133/1:6–9

Axel L (1980) Cerebral blood flow determination by rapid-sequence computed tomography: theoretical analysis. Radiology 137:679–686

Axel L, Moss AA, Berninger W (1981) Dynamic computed tomography demonstration of hepatic arteriovenous fistula. J Comput Assist Tomogr 5/1:95–98

Baert AL (1981) Dynamic scanning of liver and pancreas. Dynamic Body CT-Scanning in Europe. Tübingen 30.–31.10.1981. CT-Sonographie 2:96–107

Baert AL, Wilms G, Marchal G, Demayer P, Desomer F (1980) Contrast enhancement by bolus technique in the CT examination of the kidney. Radiologe 20:279–287

Baert AL, Usewils R, Wilms G, Marchal G, Ponette E (1981) Dynamic studies of the pancreas. In: Felix R, Katber E, Wegener OH (eds) Contrast media in computed tomography. Excerpta Medica, Amsterdam

Barnett PH, Zerhouni EA, Waite RI, Siegelman SS (1980) Computed tomography in the diagnosis of cavernous hemangioma of the liver. AJR 134:439–447

Baron RL, Gutierrez FR, Sagel SS, Levitt RG, McKnight RC (1981) CT of anomalies of the mediastinal vessels. AJR 137:571–576

Berland LL, Lawson TL, Foley WD, Melrose B, Chintapalli K, Taylor A (1982) Comparison of pre- and postcontrast CT in hepatic masses. AJR 138:853–858

Berninger WH, Reddington RW, Doherty PW, Lipton MJ, Carlsson E (1979) Gated cardiac scanning: Canine studies. J Comput Assist Tomogr 3 (2):155–163

Berninger W, Redington R, Level W et al. (1981) Technical aspects and clinical applications of CT/X, a dynamic CT scanner. J Comput Assist Tomogr 5:206–215

Brady TJ, Goldmann MR, Pykett IL et al. (1982) Proton nuclear magnetic resonance imaging of regionally ischemic canine hearts: Effects of paramagnetic proton signal enhancement. Radiology 144:343–347

Brandfonbrener M, Langdowne M, Shuck NW (1955) Changes in cardiac output with age. Circulation 12:557–566

Brasch RU (1980) Allergic reactions to contrast media: Accumulated evidence. AJR 134:797–801

Breimann R, Castellino R, Harrell G, Marshall W, Glatstein E, Kaplan H (1978) CT-pathologic correlations in Hodgkin's disease and non-Hodgkin's lymphoma. Radiology 126:159–166

Breit A, Rohde U (1979) Computertomographie in der Gynäkologie. Med Klin 74:1881

Brody WR, Enzmann DR, Deutsch LS, Hall A, Pelc N (1981) Intravenous carotid arteriography using line-scanned digital radiography. Radiology 139:297–300

Brown WH, Pearce L (1923) Studies based on a malignant tumor of the rabbit. 1. The spontaneous tumor and associated abnormalitites. J Exp Med 37:601–630

Brundage BH, Lipton MJ, Herfkens RJ, Berninger WH, Redington RW, Chatterjee K, Carlsson E (1980) Detection of patent coronary bypass grafts by CT. Circulation 61/4:826–831

Buck J, Binder JP (1982) Nachweis des Insulinoms im Pankreas durch die Röntgen-Computertomographie. Radiologe 22:279–282

Buck J, Menck F, Both A, Seitz KM (1983) Informationswert der Röntgen-Computertomographie bei Vorhoftumoren des Herzens. RöFo 1:36–41
Burgener FA, Hamlin DJ (1981) Contrast enhancement in abdominal CT: Bolus vs. infusion. AJR 6/ 137:351–358
Burgener FA, Violante MR (1979) Comparison of hepatic VX2-carcinomas after intraarterial, intraportal and intraparenchymal tumor cell injection. An angiographic and computed tomographic study in the rabbit. Invest Radiol 14:410–414

Carlsson E, Lipton MJ, Skiöldebrand CG, Berninger WH, Redington RW (1980) Erfahrungen mit der Computertomographie bei der In-vivo-Herzdiagnostik. Radiologe 20:44–49
Caron-Poitreau C, Dauver A, Vialle M, Friess JJ, Rieux D (1981) Apport de la tomodensitométrie dans le diagnostic des suppurations abdominales. J Radiol 62/5:283–290
Casarella WJ, Knowles DM, Wolf M, Johnson PM (1978) Focal nodular hyperplasia and liver cell adenoma: radiologic and pathologic differentiation. AJR 131:393–402
Castellino R, Silverman J, Gladstein E, Blank N, Wexler L (1972) Splenic arteriography in Hodgkin's disease: a roentgenologic-pathologic study of 33 consecutive untreated patients. AJR 114:574–582
Claussen CD, Singer R (1979) Progress in the diagnosis of cranio-facial injuries and tumours by computer tomography. J Maxillofac Surg 7:210–217
Claussen CD, Rinck P, Baldauf G, Pager P (1980) Zur Differentialdiagnose von Lungenrundherden der M. Rendu-Osler-Weber, A.-V. Shunts in der Lunge. Rontgenblätter 33:355–362
Claussen CD, Wegener OH, Pfister M (1981) Pancreatic cancer – Computed tomography versus ultrasound and conventional techniques. In: Husband I (ed) CT in oncology. Churchill & Livingstone, London
Claussen CD, Linke G, Felix R, Lochner B, Weinmann HJ, Wegener OH (1982a) Bolusgeometrie und -dynamik nach intravenöser Kontrastmittelinjektion. RöFo 137/2:212–216
Claussen CD, Banzer D, Schmiedel R, Lochner B (1982b) Diagnostik des Aortenaneurysmas. Dtsch Med Wochenschr 107/10:370–374
Claussen CD, Lochner B, Köhler D, Banzer D (1982c) Dynamische Computertomographie bei Gesichtsschädeltumoren. RöFo 136/2:144–150
Claussen CD, Köhler D, Schartl M, Felix R (1983a) Computertomographische und echokardiographische Diagnostik intrakardialer Raumforderungen. RöFo 138/3:296–301
Claussen CD, Weinmann HJ, Schnoy N (1983b) Tierexperimentelle Studien zum Einsatz der dynamischen Computertomographie bei Lebertumoren. RöFo 139/3:266–268
Cohen, Z, Seltzer SE, Dais MA, Hanson RN (1981) Iodinated starch particles: A new contrast material for computed tomography of the liver. J Comput Assist Tomogr 5/6:843–846
Cubilla AL, Fostner J, Fitzgerald PI (1978) Lymph node involvement in carcinoma of the head of the pancreas area. Cancer 41:880–887

Dean PB (1980) Contrast media in body computed tomography: Experimental and theoretical background, present limitations, and proposals for improved diagnostic efficacy. Invest Radiol 15:164–170
Dean PB, Kormano M (1977) Intra-arterial bolus of 125 J labelled meglumine diatrizoate: Early extravascular distribution. Acta Radiol [Diagn] (Stockh) 18:425–432
Dean PB, Kivisaari L, Kormano M (1978) The diagnostic potential of contrast enhancement pharmacokinetics. Invest Radiol 13:533–540
Dean P, Violante MR, Mahowey JA (1980) Hepatic CT contrast enhancement: Effect of dose, duration of infusion, and time elapsed following infusion. Invest Radiol 15:158–161
Dobben GD, Valvassori GE, Mafee MF, Berninger WH (1979) Evaluation of brain circulation by rapid rotational computed tomography. Radiology 133:105–111
Döhring W, Linke G (1979) Die Grundlagen der quantitativen pulmonalen Computertomographie. RöFo 130/2:133–143
Doppman JL, Rienmüller R, Lissner J, Cyran J, Bolte HD, Strauer BE, Hellwig H (1981) Computed tomography in constrictive pericardial disease. J Comput Assist Tomogr 5 (1):1–11
Drayer BP, Heinz ER, Dujovny M, Wolfson SK, Gur D (1979) Patterns of brain perfusion: Dynamic computed tomography using intravenous contrast enhancement. J Comput Assist Tomogr 3:633–640

Dunnick NR, Ihde DC, Doppman JL, Bates HR (1980) Computed tomography in primary hepatocellular carcinoma. J Comput Assist Tomogr 4/1:59–62

Egan TJ, Neiman HL, Herman RJ, Malve SR, Sanders JH (1980) Computed tomography in the diagnosis of aortic aneurysm dissection or traumatic injury. Radiology 136:141
Elke M (1982) Kontrastmittel in der Röntgendiagnostik. Thieme, Stuttgart

Felix R, Lackner K, Thurn P (1980) Derzeitige und künftige Möglichkeiten des CT-Einsatzes am Herzen. Radiologe 20:50–55
Felix R, Kazner E, Wegener OH (eds) (1981) Contrast media in computed tomography. Excerpta Medica, Amsterdam
Ferruci JT, Wittenberg J, Black EB, Kirkpatrick RH, Hall DA (1979) Computed body tomography in chronic pancreatitis. Radiology 130:175–182
Fischer HW, Morris TW (1980) Possible factors in intravascular contrast media toxicity. Invest Radiol 15:232–238
Freeny PC, Marks WM (1983) Computed tomographic arteriography of the liver. Radiology 148:193–197
Freeny PC, Vimont TR, Barnett DV (1979) Cavernous hemangioma of the liver: Ultrasonography, arteriography, and computed tomography. Radiology 132:143–148
Fretz C, Haertel M (1981) Computertomographie nach Nierentrauma. RöFo 135/6:653–656
Friedmann G, Bücheler E, Thurn P (eds) (1981) Ganzkörper-Computertomographie. Thieme, Stuttgart
Frommhold W, Hausdörfer J (1976) Hinweise zur Behandlung von Kontrastmittelzwischenfällen. Schering, Berlin
Fuchs AB (1981) Contrast enhancement in body computerized tomography. 11th Intern Symposium, Bern. Thieme and Stratton, Stuttgart NewYork
Fuchs WA, Vock P, Haertel M (1979) Pharmakokinetik intravasaler Kontrastmittel bei der Computer-Tomographie. Radiologe 19:90–93

Gado MH, Phelps ME, Coleman RE (1975) An extravascular component of contrast enhancement in cranial computed tomography, Part I, II. Radiology 117:589–597
Galanski M, Cramer RM, Drewes G (1980) Möglichkeiten der Kontrastmittelanwendung bei der Computertomographie. RöFo 132/2:139–144
Gardeur D, Lantron J, Millard JC, Berger N, Metzger J (1980) Pharmacokinetics of contrast media: Experimental results in dog and man with CT implications. J Comput Assist Tomogr 4/2:178–185
Gazer GM, Axel L, Goldberg HI, Mos AA (1981) Dynamic CT of the normal spleen. AJR 137: 343–346
Georgi M, Weiss H, Trede M, Sager HD, Bleyl U, Mittelstaedt G von (1982) Radiologische Differentialdiagnostik zystischer Nebennierenprozesse. RöFo 137/6:637–646
Godwin JD, Webb WR (1981) Dynamic computed tomography in the evaluation of vascular lung lesions. Radiology 138:629–635
Godwin JD, Herfkens RL, Skiöldebrand CG, Federle MP, Lipton MJ (1980) Evaluation of dissections and aneurysms of the thoracic aorta by conventional and dynamic CT scanning. Radiology 136:125
Godwin JD, Herfkens RJ, Skiöldebrand CG, Brundlage BH, Schiller NB, Lipton MJ (1981) Detection of intraventricular thrombi by computed tomography. Radiology 138:717–721
Gomes MN, Hakkal G, Schellinger D (1978) Ultrasonography and CT scanning. A comparative study of abdominal aortic aneurysms. Comput Tomogr 2:99
Grabbe E, Heller M (1982) Serien-Computertomographie der Leber – Möglichkeiten und Grenzen der Methode. Rontgenblätter 35:181–186
Grabbe E, Jend HH (1982) Arteriovenöse Fisteln in der Leber. RöFo 136/4:386–390
Grabbe E, Dammann HG, Heller H (1982) Wert der Computertomographie für die Prognose der akuten Pankreatitis. RöFo 136/5:534–537
Graen J, Döhring W, Grote W (1981) Angiographische und computertomographische Diagnostik von Aortenaneurysmen. RöFo 134:273
Grainger RG (1981) Formulation and clinical introduction of low osmolality contrast media. Radiology 21:261–267

Greene HSN (1949) Heterologous transplantation of the Brown-Pearce tumor. Cancer Res 9:728–735
Gross SC, Barr J, Eyler WR, Khaja F, Goldstein S (1980) Computed tomography in dissection of the thoracic aorta. Radiology 136:135
Günther R, Kümmerle F, Beyer J, Klose K, Kuhn FB, Rückert K, Cordes U (1981) Lokalisationsdiagnostik von Inselzelltumoren durch Sonographie, Computertomographie, Arteriographie und selektive Hormonbestimmung. RöFo 135/6: 657–662

Hacker H, Becker H (1977) Time contolled computed tomographic angiography. J Comput Assist Tomogr 1/4:405–409
Haertel M (1980) Das kavernöse Leberhämangiom im Computertomogramm. RöFo 133/4:379–381
Haertel M, Tillmann V, Fuchs WA (1979) Die akute Pankreatitis im Computertomogramm. RöFo 130/5:525–530
Haertel M, Zaunbauer W, Fuchs WA (1980) Die computertomographische Morphologie des Pankreaskarzinoms. RöFo 133/1:1–5
Hamlin DJ, Burgener FA, Beecham JB (1981) CT of intramural endometrial carcinoma: Contrast enhancement is essential. AJR 137:551–554
Harris RD, Usselman JA, Vinton CV, Warmath MA (1979) Computerized tomographic diagnosis of aneurysms of the thoracic aorta. Comput Tomogr 3:879
Havron A, Davis MA, Seltzer SE, Paskins-Hurlburt AI, Hessel SI (1980) Heavy metal particulate contrast material for computed tomography of the liver. J Comput Assist Tomogr 4/5:642–648
Hayman LA, Evans RA, Hinck VC (1979) Rapid high dose (RHD) contrast cranial computed tomography – A concise review of normal anatomy. J Comput Assist Tomogr 3:147–154
Hegglin R, Rutishauser W, Kaufmann G, Luethy E, Scheu H (1962) Kreislaufdiagnostik mit der Farbstoffverdünnungsmethode. Thieme, Stuttgart
Heiberg E, Wolberson M, Sundaram M, Connors J, Susman W (1981) CT findings in thoracic aortic dissection. AJR 136:13
Heinz ER, Dubois P, Osborne D, Drayer B, Barrett W (1979) Dynamic computed tomography study of the brain. J Comput Assist Tomogr 3 (5):641–549
Heinz ER, Dubois PJ, Drayer BP, Hill R (1980) A preliminary investigation of the role of dynamic computed tomography in renovascular hypertension. J Comput Assist Tomogr 4/1:63–66
Heinz ER, Fram E, Johanson GA, Godwin D (1982) Dynamic scanning. In: Lissner J, Doppman JL (eds) CT'82 Internationales Computertomographie Symposium, Seefeld/Tirol 28.–30. Januar 1982. Schnetztor, Konstanz
Heller M, Gürtler KF, Grabbe E (1981a) Seriencomputertomographie. In: Friedmann G, Bücheler E, Thurn P (eds) Ganzkörpercomputertomographie. Thieme, Stuttgart
Heller M, Grabbe E, Bücheler E (1981b) Serien-Computertomographie – Methodik und erste Erfahrungen. RöFo 134/1:16–21
Heller M, Jend HH, Grabbe E, Hambüchen K (1981c) Seriencomputertomographie. Electromedica 2:68–73
Heller M, Huland H, Hagemann J, Bischoff K (1981d) Computertomographische Diagnostik von renalen und extrarenalen Komplikationen bei Nierentransplantaten – „statische" und „dynamische" Untersuchungen. Comput Tomogr 1:184–192
Heller M, Guthoff R, Hagemann J, Jend HH (1982) CT of malignant choroidal melanoma – Morphology and perfusion characteristics. Neuroradiology 23:23–30
Henegham MA, Biancaniello TM, Heidelberger E, Peterson SB, Marsh MJ, Lauterbur PC (1982) Nuclear magnetic resonance zeugmatographic imaging of the heart: Application to the study of ventricular septal defect. Radiology 143:183–186
Herman RE, Cooperman AM (1979) Current concepts in cancer. Cancer of the pancreas. N Engl J Med 301/9:482–485
Herms HJ (1978) Kontastmittel – Anforderungen, Möglichkeiten, Risiken. Neuroradiology 16: 482–486
Heuck F, Anschütz F, Schwarzkopf HJ (1963) Ein röntgenkinematographisches Verfahren zur quantitativen Bestimmung des Blutvolumens. RöFo 98/4:428:438
Heuck F, Vanselow K (1970) Methodik und Möglichkeiten einer densitometrischen Kreislaufanalyse. RöFo 112/1:69–83

Heuser L, Friedmann G (1982) Technik der Kontrastmittelapplikation bei der Computertomographie des Herzens. Radiologe 22:26–31
Heuser L, Friedman CG, Mödder U (1978) Computer-tomographischer Nachweis der Aorten-Aneurysmen. Radiologe 18:482
Heuser L, Lackner K, Hauser H (1982) Validität der Computertomographie bei der Darstellung offener und verschlossener aortokoronarer Venenbrücken (ACVB). RöFo 137/6:619–626
Hidalgo H, Korobkin M, Breiman RS, Kisslo JR (1981) CT of intracardiac tumor. AJR 137: 608–609
Higgins CB, Sovak M, Schmidt W, Siemers PR (1978) Uptake of contrast materials by experimental acute myocardial infarctions: A preliminary report. Invest Radiol 13:337–339
Hindel R (1982) Probleme bei der Datenauswertung von dynamischen CT-Aufnahmen. Röntgenpraxis 35:329–331
Hosoki T, Chantani M, Mori S (1982) Dynamic computed tomography of hepatocellular carcinoma. AJR 139:1099–1106
Hounsfield GN (1973) Computerized transverse axial scanning (tomography). Part I. Description of system. Br J Radiol 46:1016–1022
Huber DJ, Lapray JF, Hessel SJ (1981) In vivo evaluation of experimental myocardial infarction by ungated CT. AJR 136:469–473
Hübener KH (1978) Computertomographische Densitometrie von Leber, Milz und Nieren bei intravenös verabreichten lebergängigen Kontrastmitteln in Bolusform. RöFo 129:289–297
Hübener KH, Klott KJ (1980) „Statisches" und dynamisches Kontrastmittelenhancement der Körperstamm-Computertomographie. RöFo 133/4:347–354
Hübener KH, Schmitt WGH (1979) Die computertomographische Diagnostik von Abszeßbildungen. RöFo 130/1:53–57
Hübener KH, Kalender WA, Metzger HOFJ (1982) Fast digital recording of X-ray dilution arves: a preliminary evaluation. Radiology 145:545–547

Inamoto K, Sugiki K, Yamasaki H, Nakao N, Miura T (1980) Computed tomography and angiography of hepatocellular carcinoma. J Comput Assist Tomogr 4/6:832–839
Ishikawa J, Onouchi Z, Saito Y, Kitada H, Shinoda A, Ushitani K, Tabuchi M, Suzuki M (1981) Renal cortex visualization and analysis of dynamic CT curves of the kidney. J Comput Assist Tomogr 5/5:695–701
Itai Y, Nishikawa J, Tasaka A (1978) Computed tomography in the evaluation of hepatocellular carcinoma. Radiology 131:165–170
Itai Y, Araki T, Yoshikawa K, Furui s, Yashirol N, Tasaka A (1980) Computed tomography of gallbladder carcinoma. Radiology 137:713–718
Itai Y, Araki T, Furui S, Tasaka A (1981) Differential diagnosis of hepatic masses on computed tomography with particular reference to hepatocellular carcinoma. J Comput Assist Tomogr 5/6:834–842
Itai Y, Moss AA, Goldberg HI (1982a) Transient hepatic attenuation difference of lobar or segmental distribution detected by dynamic computed tomography. Radiology 144:835–839
Itai Y, Araki T, Tasaka T, Maruyama M (1982b) Computed tomographic appearance of resectable pancreatic carcinoma. Radiology 143:719–726
Itai Y, Araki T, Furui S et al. (1983) Computed tomography of primary intrahepatic biliary malignancy. Radiology 147:485–490
Itzchak Y, Groszmann RJ, Glickman MG (1978) The effect of hepatic arterial injection of contrast medium, blood, and saline on hepatic artery flow. Invest Radiol 6:528–532

Johnson CM, Sheedy PF, Stanson AW, Stephens DH, Haltery RR, Adson MA (1981) Computed tomography and angiography of cavernous hemangiomas of the liver. Radiology 138:115–121
Johnson GA, Godwin JO, Fram EV (1982) Gated multiplanar cardiac computed tomography. Radiology 145:195–197

Kahl FR, Wolfman NT, Watts LE (1981) Evaluation of aortocoronary bypass graft status by computed tomography. Am J Cardiol 48:304–310
Kalender WA (1981) Current CT technology for dynamic CT application: Limitations and future perspectives. Dynamic Body-CT Scanning in Europe, Tübingen 30.–31.10.1981. CT-Sonographie 2:96–107

Kirkpatrick JB (1978) The blood-brain barrier. Its role in contrast studies. Comput Tomogr 2: 189–196
Kirschner H, Burmester U, Stringaris K (1977) CT-Tomometrie Teil 2: Diagnostik jodhaltiger Kontrastmittel. Strahlentherapie 153:616–619
Kirschner H, Krempl A, Poppe H (1981) Die Häufigkeit von Nebenwirkungen während der zweiphasigen Bolusperfusion und der einphasigen Bolusinjektion eines renalen Röntgenkontrastmittels in der abdominellen Computertomographie. Comput Tomogr 1:155–171
Kivisaari L, Kormano M, Rantakouko V (1979) Contrast enhancement of the pancreas in computed tomography. J Comput Assit Tomogr 3:722–726
Kleinhaus U, Goldsher D, Kaftori JK (1982) Computed tomographic diagnosis of abdominal abscesses. Radiologe 22:230–234
Knöfel PK, Kraft RP, Knight RD, Moore SK (1974) Sodium versus meglumine diatrizoate in excretory urography. Invest Radiol 9:117
König R, Herter M (1983) Zur Differentialdiagnostik benigner intrahepatischer Raumforderungen. RöFo 138/1:1–7
Kormano MJ (1981) Kinetics of contrast media after bolus injection and infusion. In: Felix R, Kazner E, Wegener OH (eds) Contrast media in computed tomography. Excerpta Medica, Amsterdam, pp 39–45
Kormano M, Dean PB (1976) Extravascular contrast material: The major component of contrast enhancement. Radiology 121:379–382
Korobkin M, Kressel HY, Moss AA, Koehler RE (1978) Computed tomographic angiography of the body. Radiology 126:807–811
Kreel L, Haertel M, Katz D (1977) Computed tomography of the normal pancreas. J Comput Ass Tomogr 1:290–299
Kruger RA, Anderson RE, Koehler PR, Nelson JA, Sorenson JA, Morgan T (1981) Method for the non-invasive evaluation of cardiovascular dynamics using a digital radiographic device. Radiology 139:301–305

Lackner K, Thurn P (1980) EKG-gesteuerte Kardiocomputertomographie. RöFo 132/2:164–169
Lackner K, Thurn P (1981) Computed tomography of the heart: ECG-gated and continuous scans. Radiology 140:413–420
Lackner K, Frommhold H, Thurn P (1979) Vergleich der Gefäßdarstellungen in Abdomen und Retroperitonealraum mit Computertomographie und Ultraschall. RöFo 131:479
Lackner K, Thurn P, Orrdano L, Schuppen V, Simon H, Kirchhoff PG (1980) Der aortokoronare Bypass im CT. RöFo 133/5:459–464
Lackner K, Hahn N, Reske SN, Eichelkraut W, Thurn P (1982) Der experimentelle Myokardinfarkt im Computertomogramm. RöFo 137/2:152–161
Ladurner G (1978) Die Bestimmung des zerebralen Blutvolumens mit der Computertomographie in grauer und weißer Substanz. Fortschr Neurol Psychiatr 46:369–381
Ladurner G, Zilkha E, Sager WD, Iliff LD, Lechner H, Du Boulay GH (1979) Measurement of regional cerebral blood volume using the EMI 1010 scanner. Br J Radiol 52:371–374
Lagemann K (1976) Pharmakokinetik angiographischer Kontrastmittel unter besonderer Berücksichtigung des extravasalen Raumes. RöFo 124/1:69–75
Lalli AF, Greenstreet R (1981) Reactions to contrast media: Testing the CNS hypothesis. Radiology 138:47–49
Lange S, Steinhoff H, Avilés C, Kazner E, Grumme T (1979) Kontrastmittelkinetik in zerebralen Tumoren. RöFo 130/6:666–669
Larde D, Belloir C, Vasile N, Frija J, Ferrane J (1980) Computed tomography of aortic dissection. Radiology 136:147
Lasser EC (1981) New aspects of contrast media reactions: Considerations, etiology, and prophylaxis. In: Felix R, Kazner E, Wegener OH (eds) Contrast media in computed tomography. Excerpta Medica, Amsterdam, p 49
Lasser EC, Lang JH, Hamblin AE, Lyon SG, Howard M (1980) Activation systems in contrast idiosyncrasy. Invest Radiol 15:52–55
Lipton JJ, Higgins CB (1980) Evaluation of ischemic heart diseases by computed tomography. Radiol Clin North Am 18/3:557–575

Lochner B, Claussen CD, Christ F, Brandt H (1982) Computertomographische Diagnostik von Ovarialtumoren. Strahlentherapie 158:659–662
Lochner B, Loddenkemper R, Claussen CD, Wegener OH (1983) Thorakoskopische und Computertomographische Befunde beim Pleuramesotheliom. RöFo 138
Love L, Churchill R, Reynes C, Schuster GA, Moncada R, Berkow A (1979) Computed tomography staging of renal carcinoma. Urol Radiol 1:3–10

Majewski A, Hendrickx P, Brölsch C, Wiese H (1983) Computertomographische Densitometrie primärer Lebertumoren. RöFo 138/1:8–14
Marchal G, Baert AL, Wilms G (1979) Intravenous pancreaticography in computed tomography. J Comput Assist Tomogr 3/6:727–732
Marchal G, Baert AL, Wilms BE (1980a) CT of noncystic liver lesions: Bolus enhancement. AJR 135:57–65
Marchal G, Wilms G, Baert A, Ponette E (1980b) Applications of specific vascular opacification in CT of the upper abdomen. RöFo 132/1:45–48
Marks WM, Jacobs RP, Goodman PC, Lim RC (1979) Hepatocellular carcinoma: clinical and angiographic findings and predictability for surgical resection. AJR 132:7–11
Matsui O, Kadoya M, Suzuki M et al. (1983) Work in progress: Dynamic sequential computed tomography during arterial portography in the detection of hepatic neoplasms. Radiology 146:721–727
Mauro MA, Wadsworth DE, Stanley RJ, McClennan BL (1982) Renal cell carcinoma: Angiography in the CT-era. AJR 139:1135–1138
Meaney TF, Randkivi U, McIntyre WJ, Gallagher JH, Haaga JR, Havrilla TR, Reich NE (1980) Detection of low-contrast lesions in computed body tomography: An experimental study of simulated lesions. Radiology 134:149–154
Mödder U, Friedmann G, Rosenberger J (1981) Wert der Angio-CT für Stadieneinteilung, Verlaufsbeobachtung und Therapie bei akuter Pankreatitis. RöFo 134/1:22–27
Moss AA, Schrumpf J, Schnyder P, Korobkin M, Shimshak RR (1979) Computed tomography of focal hepatic lesions: a blind clinical evaluation of the effect of contrast enhancement. Radiology 131:427–430
Moss AA, Dean PB, Goldberg HJ (1982) Dynamic CT of hepatic masses with intravenous and intraarterial contrast material. AJR 138:847–852
Müller HA, van Kaick G, Schaaf J, Lüllig H, Vogt-Moykopf I, Delphendahl A (1981) Präoperatives Stagung des Bronchialkarzinoms: Wertigkeit der Computertomographie im Vergleich zur konventionellen Radiologie. RöFo 134/6:601–607
Mützel W (1981a) Properties of conventional contrast media. In: Felix R, Kazner E, Wegener OH (eds) Contrast media in computed tomography. Excerpta Medica, Amsterdam, pp 19–26
Mützel W (1981b) Distribution dynamics of contrast media. Dynamic body CT-scanning in Europe. Tübingen, 30.–31.10.1981. CT-Sonographie 2:96–107

Naidich DP, McCauley DI, Khouri NF et al. (1983) Computed tomography of lobar collapse: 1. Endobronchial obstruction. J Comput Assist Tomogr 7/5:745–757
Nair CK, Sketch MH, Mahoney PD, Lynch JD, Mouss AN, Kenney NP (1981) Detection of left ventricular thrombi by computerized tomography. Br Heart J 45:535–541
Nakao N, Miura K, Takayasu Y et al. (1983) CT angiography in hepatocellular carcinoma. J Comput Assist Tomogr 7/5:780–787
Newell JD, Higgins CB, Abraham JL, Kelley MJ, Schmidt WS, Haigler F (1980) Computerized tomographic appearance of evolving myocardial infarctions. Invest Radiol 15:207–214
Newhouse JH, Murphy RX (1981) Tissue distribution of soluble contrast: Effect of dose variation and chances with time. AJR 136:463–467
Nino-Murcia M, Kurtz A, Brennan RE et al. (1983) CT diagnosis of an artery pseudoaneurysm: A complication of chronic pancreatitis and pseudocyst formation. J Comput Assist Tomogr 7/5: 527–529
Nishikawa J, Itai Y, Tasaka A (1981) Lobar attenuation of the liver on computed tomography. Radiology 141:725–728
Norman D, Stevens EA, Wing SD, Levin V, Newton TH (1978) Quantitative aspects of contrast enhancement in cranial computed tomography. Radiology 129:683–688

Norman D, Axel L, Berninger WH, Edwards MS, Cann CE, Redington RW, Cox L (1981) Dynamic computed tomography of the brain: Techniques, data analysis, and applications. AJR 136: 759–770

Ono N, Martinez CR, Fara JW, Hodges FJ (1980) Diatrizoate distribution in dogs as a function of administration rate and time following intravenous injection. J Comput Assist Tomogr 4:174–177

Pedrosa CS, Casnova R, Lezana AH, Fernandez MC (1981) Computed tomography in obstructive jaundice, Part II. Radiology 139:635–645

Piekarski J, Goldberg HI, Royal SA, Axel L, Moss AA (1980a) Difference between liver and spleen CT numbers in the normal adult: its usefulness in predicting the presence of diffuse liver disease. Radiology 137:727–729

Piekarski J, Federle M, Moss A, London S (1980b) Computed tomography of the spleen. Radiology 135:683–689

Prando A, Wallce S, Bernardino ME, Lindell MM (1979) Computed tomographic arteriography of the liver. Radiology 130:697–701

Pullicino P, Kendall BE (1980) Contrast enhancement in ischaemic lesions I. Relationship to prognosis. Neuroradiology 19:235–239

Rienmüller R, Lissner J, Kment A et al. (1982) Das enddiastolische Volumen des linken Ventrikels in der Computertomographie im Vergleich zur Herzkatheterventrikulographie. Comput Tomogr 1:62–67

Ring J (1979) Die Problematik der Kontrastmittelüberempfindlichkeit. Dtsch Med Wochenschr 104:517–524

Rogers JV, Mack LA, Freeny PC, Johnson ML, Sones PJ (1981) Hepatic focal nodular hyperplasia: Angiography, CT, sonography, and scintigraphy. AJR 137:983–990

Rohde U, Steinbrich W, Friedmann G (1982) Computertomographie der Ovarialtumoren – Fortschritte in der Diagnostik. Radiologe 22:146

Rossi P, Rovighi L, Tipaldi L, Bompiari C, Simonetti G (1981) High contrast enhancement of the liver in CT by repeated doses of contrast medium. Eur J Radiol 1:126–131

Sager WD, Stöffler F, Ladurner G, zur Nedden D, Hammer B (1982) Statische und dynamische Kontrastmittelverwendung in der cranialen Computertomographie. In: Lissner J, Doppman JL (eds) CT'82 Internationales Computertomographie Symposium. Seefeld/Tirol 28.–30. 1. 1982. Schnetztor, Konstanz

Schad N, Schepke P, Rohde U, Schepke H, Schmid V (1981) Timing of exposure in angiographic computed tomography. Cardiovasc Intervent Radiol 4:59–65

Schatz M, Patterson R, Orourke J, Nickelsen J, Northup C (1975) The administration of radiographic contrast media to patients with a history of previous reaction. J Allerg Clin Immunol 55:358–366

Scheid KF, Lissner J, Blaha H, Gebauer A (1981) Densitometrische Analyse pulmonaler Rundherde im Computertomogramm. RöFo 134/4:357–363

Scherer V, Lissner J, Brall B, Eisenburg J, Zrenner M, Schildberg FW (1979) Computertomographie der Leber. RöFo 130/5:531–535

Schittenhelm R, Schwierz G (1981) Technik und Bildaufbau. In: Friedmann G, Bückeler E, Thurn P (Hrsg) Ganzkörpercomputertomographie. Thieme, Stuttgart, pp 1–39

Schröder J, Keller H, Terwey B, Mittmann V (1981) Hämodynamische Effekte der intraarteriellen Kontrastmittelinjektion. RöFo 135/2:143–151

Schultz E, Felix R (1978) I. Phantommessungen zum räumlichen Auflösungsvermögen und zum Partial-Volume-Effect bei der Computertomographie. RöFo 129/6:673–678

Schultz E, Lackner K (1981) Die Auswirkung von Strahlenschwächung und Strahlenaufhärtung auf die gemessenen CT-Werte. Comput Tomogr 1:83–88

Schultz E, Felix R, Lackner K, Bergeder HD, Thurn P (1979) II. Räumliches Auflösungsvermögen, Dichteauflösung und Partial-Volume-Effekt bei kugelförmigen Objekten verschiedenen Durchmessers. RöFo 130/4:479–486

Selzer A, Dunlap RW, Wray HW, Russel J (1968) A critical appraisal of the circulation time test. Arch Intern Med 122:491–495

Sheedy PF, Stephens DH, Hattery RR, MacCarty RL (1977) Computed tomography in the evaluation of patients with suspected carcinoma of the pancreas. Radiology 124:731–737
Shehadi WH (1975) Adverse reactions to intravascularly administered contrast media. AJR 124: 145–152
Shehadi WH, Toniolo G (1980) Adverse reactions to contrast media. Radiology 137:299–302
Sommer B, Doppman JL, Stelter W, Mayr M, Rienmüller R, Lissner J (1981) Der diagnostische Stellenwert der Computertomographie bei mediastinalen Erkrankungen in Abhängigkeit von deren Lokalisation. Comput Tomogr 1:35–42
Speck V, Nagel R, Leistenschneider W, Mützel W (1977) Pharmakokinetik und Biotransformation neuer Röntgenkontrastmittel für die Uro- und Angiographie beim Patienten. RöFo 127/3: 270–274
Stieve FE, Schmidt T (1981) Strahlenexposition und Strahlenschutz bei der Computertomographie. Rontgenpraxis 34:87–97
Sutton P, Al-Kutoubi MA, Lipkin DP (1982) Left atrial myxoma diagnosed by computerized tomography. Br J Radiol 55:81–84

Tada S, Fukuda K, Aoyagi Y, Hareda J (1980) CT of abdominal malignancies: Dynamic approach. AJR 135:455–461
Taenzer V, Albrecht A, Clauß W, Held J (1981) Natrium- oder Methylglukaminsalze der Kontrastmittel für die Infusionsurographie? Radiologe 21:288–290
Thomas JL, Bernardino ME, Vermess M et al. (1982) EOE-13 in the detection of hepatosplenic lymphoma. Radiology 145:629–634
Tomoda H, Mitsumoto H, Furuya H, Shotsu A, Outaki M, Matsuyama S (1981) Evaluation of left ventricular thrombus with computed tomography. Am J Cardiol 48:573–577
Traupe H, Heiss WD, Hoeffken W, Zülch KJ (1979) Hyperperfusion and enhancement in dynamic computed tomography of ischemic stroke patients. J Comput Assist Tomogr 3:629–632
Traupe H, Heiss WD, Hoeffken W, Zülch KJ (1980) Perfusion patterns in CT transit studies. Neuroradiology 19:181–191
Treugut H, Nyman U, Hildell J (1980) Sequenz-CT: Frühe Dichteveränderungen der gesunden Niere nach Kontrastmittelapplikation. Radiologe 20:558–562
Treugut H, Nyman U, Hildell J, Molde A (1981a) Funktionskontrolle des Nierentransplantats durch Sequenz-CT – Erste Ergebnisse. RöFo 135/2:133–142
Treugut H, Anderson I, Hildell J, Nyman U, Weibull H (1981b) Diagnostik renaler Perfusionsstörungen durch Sequenz-CT. RöFo 135/4:381–388
Tschakert H (1980) Zeitlicher Ablauf des Dichteverhaltens von Lebermetastasen nach Kontrastmittelgabe. RöFo 133/2:171–176

Vermess M, Adamson RH, Doppman JL, Girton M (1977) Computed tomographic demonstration of hepatic tumor with the aid of intravenous iodinated fat emulsion. Radiology 125:711–715
Vermess M, Chattery DC, Doppman JL, Grimes G, Adamson RH (1979) Development and experimental evaluation of a contrast medium for computed tomographic examination of the liver and spleen. J Comput Assist Tomogr 3/1:25–31
Violante MR, Dean PB (1980) Improved detectability of VX2 carcinoma in the rabbit liver with contrast enhancement in computed tomography. Radiology 134:237–239
Vock P, Tillmann U, Fuchs WA (1981) Computertomographie des Mediastinums. Radiologe 21: 336–336

Walter E, Hübener KH (1980) Computertomographische Charakteristika raumfordernder Prozesse im vorderen Mediastinum und ihre Differentialdiagnose. RöFo 133/4:391–400
Watanabe TJ, LaMasters D, Turski PA, Newton TH (1982) Contrast enhancement of the normal orbit. In: Felix R, Kazner E, Wegener OH (eds) Contrast media in computed tomography. International Workshop Berlin, January 1981. Excerpta Medica, Amsterdam
Wegener OH (1980a) Kontrastmittel in der Computertomographie. Schering, Berlin
Wegener OH (1980b) Artefakte in der Computertomographie. RöFo 132/6:643–651
Wegener OH (1981) Ganzkörpercomputertomographie. Karger, München

Wegener OH, Claussen CD (1981) Contrast media in computed tomography of the mediastinum and the lung. In: Felix R, Kazner E, Wegener OH (eds) Contrast media in computed tomography. Excerpta Medica, Amsterdam, pp 214–221
Wegener OH, Mützel W, Souchon R (1980) Contrast media for computer tomography of the liver. Acta Radiol [Diagn] (Stockh) 21:239–247
Weinmann HJ, Mützel W, Souchon R, Wegener OH (1981) Experimental water-soluble contrast media for computed tomography of the liver. In: Felix R, Kazner E, Wegener OH (eds) Contrast media in computed tomography. Excerpta Media, Amsterdam, pp 95–100
Wende S, Speck U (1981) Das Kontrastmittel-Risiko bei der Computertomographie. Radiologe 21:268–273
Weymann PJ, McClennan BL, Stanley RJ, Levitt RG, Sagel SS (1980) Comparison of computed tomography and angiography in the evaluation of renal cell carcinoma. Radioloy 137:417–424
Wing DS, Anderson E, Osborn AG (1980) Dynamic cranial computed tomography. Preliminary results. Am J Roentgenol 134:941–945
Wing SD, Anderson RE, Osborn AG (1982) Cranial computed angiotomography. Radiology 143:103–107
Winkler EA (1981) Zur Problematik der angiographischen Differentialdiagnose zwischen Hypernephrom, Angiomyolipom und Nierenbeckenkarzinom. Röntgenblätter 34:133–138
Witten DM, Hirsch FD, Hartman GW (1973) Acute reactions to urographic contrast medium; incidence, clinical characteristics and relationship to history of hypersensitivity states. AJR 119:832–840

Young SW, Turner RJ, Castellino RA (1980a) A strategy for the contrast enhancement of malignant tumors using dynamic computed tomography and intravascular pharmacokinetics. Radiology 137:137–147
Young SW, Noon MA, Nassi M, Castellino RA (1980b) Dynamic computed tomography body scanning. J Comput Assist Tomogr 4/7:168–173
Young SW, Muller H, Marincek B (1981a) Contrast enhancement of malignant tumors after intravenous polyvinylpyrrolidone with metallic salts as determined by computed tomography. Radiology 138:97–105
Young SW, Noon MA, Marincek B (1981b) Dynamic computed tomography time-density study of normal human tissue after intravenous contrast administration. Invest Radiol 16:36–39

Zoneveld FW (1980) Computed tomography. Philips, Eindhoven

Subject Index

MIX
Papier aus verantwortungsvollen Quellen
Paper from responsible sources
FSC® C105338

If you have any concerns about our products,
you can contact us on
ProductSafety@springernature.com

In case Publisher is established outside the EU,
the EU authorized representative is:
Springer Nature Customer Service Center GmbH
Europaplatz 3, 69115 Heidelberg, Germany

Printed by Libri Plureos GmbH
in Hamburg, Germany